M.E.
AND YOU

**A self-help plan for managing
Myalgic Encephalomyelitis**
(known in America as Chronic Fatigue Syndrome)
**and improving the quality
of your life**

About the author

Steve Wilkinson writes from personal experience. In 1986 he became a victim of the debilitating disease myalgic encephalo-myelitis (M.E.), although it was not diagnosed as such for many months.

Always a strong advocate of self-help, he has managed, through the use of various alternative therapies, to restore his health to the extent that he is now largely able to live and work as normal.

He works from his home in south-east London as a writer and a healer, and he continues to conduct research with other sufferers into ways in which M.E. can be alleviated.

M.E.
AND YOU

A SURVIVOR'S GUIDE TO
POST-VIRAL FATIGUE SYNDROME

Steve Wilkinson

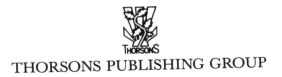
THORSONS PUBLISHING GROUP

First published 1988

British Library Cataloguing in Publication Data

Wilkinson, Steve
M.E. and you.
1. Man. Myalgic encephalomyelitis
I. Title
616.8'3

ISBN 0-7225-1802-1

Published by Thorsons Publishers Limited,
Wellingborough, Northamptonshire NN8 2RQ, England

Printed and bound in Great Britain by
Mackays of Chatham PLC, Chatham, Kent

9   10   8

Dedication

To Les and Gloria Wilkinson
with thanks for their constant love and support

Contents

1 M.E. and me: a personal introduction   9
2 The disease . . .   19
3 . . . and its symptoms   27
4 The treatment   48
5 M.A. beats M.E.: the importance of
    mental attitude   91
6 For the carers   101
   Useful addresses   106
   Further reading   109
   Index   110

1

M.E. AND ME:
A personal introduction

Like many people, I gained my first awareness of M.E. via the newspapers. It was being called 'the Yuppie disease' or 'Yuppie flu' in the tabloids, and was reported almost as a comic story. The writers took the attitude that sufferers were well-off but work-shy neurotics, and implied that the illness was a fashionable excuse for doing as little as possible. This attitude, while being very harsh on the sufferers, was quite understandable. At that time most doctors felt the same way and were inclined to refer their M.E. patients for psychiatric treatment rather than accept that they might have a genuine, physically based illness.

Happily, over the years I have cultivated a healthy scepticism about everything I read in the papers, and I have worked in the alternative health field for long enough to know that orthodox medicine is far from having all of the answers about health and well-being. When, in the course of my work, I met patients whose symptoms suggested the Yuppie disease, I was able to approach their problem with an open mind.

It soon became clear to me that this was no imaginary illness. By talking to as many sufferers as I could find, along with their families and friends, I discovered that each patient experienced the same basic symptoms. If they had all been neurotic or hysterical, as the doctors tended to think, then there would not have been these widespread similarities between patients. Also, most of the people I saw were obviously well balanced emotionally and socially, and they had all been physically and mentally healthy until the illness struck. These facts convinced me that the illness had a physical origin rather than a mental one.

Once I was satisfied in my own mind that the illness was

organic, and not evidence of some psychosomatic disorder, I began to explore various methods of treatment. The patients I had contacted during my investigations were happy to try alternative therapies because there was then, and is now, no orthodox treatment available. With my encouragement and advice they experimented with different therapies, and almost all of them found a treatment which helped them to live and work as normal.

Then, as other projects came up and the emphasis of my work altered, I gradually lost touch with the Yuppie disease and its sufferers. By this time the newspapers had started calling it 'post-viral fatigue syndrome', and reporting it as a serious illness. This new respect from the media came about because the evidence that the illness had a physical cause was growing fast as more doctors and scientists started looking into it.

In the spring of the following year I caught a nasty low-grade flu virus, and spent a couple of weeks feeling miserable. With the perfect vision of hindsight, I now know that this was probably the first intrusion of the M.E. virus into my system. At the time, it did not occur to me to consider it as anything worse than flu. I soon discovered my mistake.

In the following weeks and months I was constantly ill, with a baffling array of symptoms. The most annoying of these was a violent, angry rash which appeared on any parts of my body exposed to the sun. The rash was ferociously itchy, and once it had appeared it grew steadily worse. From small red pin-pricks it developed into large swollen bumps which split and cracked. My doctor told me that it was prickly heat, which rather surprised me. Prickly heat is a rash caused by the salt in sweat irritating the skin as the sweat evaporates. My surprise was due to the fact that most of the time I was feeling extremely cold; I spent much of the summer bundled up in sweaters in an effort to keep warm. I simply was not sweating to any noticeable degree. Also, I was weak and tired the whole time, and frequently confused and depressed. It seemed rather optimistic to assume that prickly heat could account for all of these symptoms. Eventually, because the broken skin became infected, I was given a course of antibiotics. These helped, but the rash persisted throughout the rest of the summer and autumn.

For a few weeks in November, everything seemed fine and I started to feel that life was returning to normal. Then, without any warning, I became severely ill. I constantly felt exhausted and deeply depressed. Weakness of the muscles and the will prevented me from doing even the simplest things for myself. I was always in pain, and cold and shivery, but at night fevers struck and my sweat soaked the bedclothes. I could not speak properly, or understand anything I saw or heard. My joints and muscles were continuously sore and stiff, and the pains in my head, neck and nerves defied description. I fell into uneasy sleeps every few hours, awakening unrefreshed. I felt sick at the thought of food and lost weight rapidly. I lost the use of my memory, often stopping dead in the middle of a sentence, forgetting everything I was about to say. To complicate matters, the glands in my neck became infected and I suffered badly from urethritis. I was in a dreadful state.

At this point my doctors declared that I was suffering from glandular fever. This seems a very odd diagnosis now, but then I simply could not think clearly enough to understand what they were saying or to question their opinion. I went along with what they said, hoping desperately to get well. Unfortunately, I got worse instead of better.

I suffered throughout the next year, especially in summer when the rash returned to add to the other difficulties. The doctors continued to treat me for glandular fever, even though three separate blood tests showed that I did not have that disease. The only treatment that had any effect whatsoever was antibiotics – I ended up taking these for over twenty weeks during that terrible year. But I certainly wouldn't recommend this since there is substantial evidence that antibiotics exacerbate M.E. and this can be very damaging in the long term.

Just as I started to think that I was never going to get well, the illness began to recede. For the first time in months I could do things for myself and take an interest in my surroundings. Most glorious of all was the fact that I could think again – I had a brain instead of wet cotton wool. I soon found out, though, that I had to be extremely careful. The slightest mental or physical exertion left me feeling awful. As soon as I felt strong enough, I searched out all of my reference books and put my newly refound brain into gear for a good hard think about what had been happening to me.

One thing was immediately obvious. I did not have glandular fever. With that out of my mind, I started to look through my notes and references to figure out exactly what had been wrong. Of course, it soon became clear that I was suffering from a classic case of post-viral fatigue syndrome, as it was then called. As I read back through my notes on the subject and on my interviews with sufferers, it was like reading a list of my own symptoms.

It was comforting to be able to put a label on my illness. It immediately became less frightening, less ominous. At the same time, it made me face up to a few hard facts: at that time no one knew what caused the illness, there was no treatment for it, and there was not even a suggestion of a cure. However, I knew from past experience that alternative therapies could help, and that sufferers could live and work largely as normal if they were sensible. Cheered by the prospect of being able to help myself, I started sorting out those therapies which seemed most suitable for me.

By begging help from friends and colleagues – masseurs, herbalists, reflexologists, healers and so on – and by putting my own skills to use, I started to try the various therapies. It was a long process. Some were obviously unsuitable and could be ruled out at once. Others were borderline cases which I felt I had to try to see if they could be helpful. Along the way there were periods of weeks, sometimes months, when the illness returned and I felt myself slipping back to square one. These were perhaps the worst times of all. It seems as though I was losing all hope as well as my fragile grasp on health. But as I sorted through the therapies and continued regularly with those that offered the most promise, a wonderful thing started to happen. The relapses became shorter and less frequent. As the periods between bouts of illness grew longer, I grew stronger. I started to believe that the therapies I had selected were eventually going to prove effective. At last I felt as though it was possible to win.

One evening my father told me about a radio programme he had been listening to. It was a medical phone-in during which a caller had described symptoms which were exactly the same as mine. The radio doctor had advised her to contact the M.E.

Association. As I had never heard of this group, I wrote to them to find out about it. In due course I received some leaflets from them. The leaflets described how the illness had been known as post-viral fatigue syndrome, and how it had now been reclassified as myalgic encephalomyelitis. Most important of all, they said that researchers had discovered the virus which causes the disease, and could now test for the presence of the virus in sufferers.

I was fairly ill at this time and seeing my doctor regularly. At my next appointment I brought up the subject of M.E. and asked for a test. The response astounded me. The doctor obviously knew nothing about myalgic encephalomyelitis, which was unfortunate but understandable. However, her attitude was that if she knew nothing about the illness, then I couldn't possibly be suffering from it. I was feeling too ill and weak to argue it out, but then and there I made up my mind to try and find a more sympathetic doctor.

Luckily I found one fairly soon. The new doctor's practice was miles away from where I lived, but the difficulties of the journey were made worthwhile when I got there. He was charming and courteous, and willing to listen to me as I described what I had been going through and explained what I thought might be the cause. He then examined me thoroughly and took several blood samples for analysis. He explained that though he thought I had M.E. he would test for several other possibilities at the same time. Greatly reassured, I left the surgery with high hopes. Two weeks later he phoned me with the test results and confirmed the diagnosis of M.E.

Even though I had been sure that this was my problem, the relief of knowing definitely was incredible. With renewed strength I returned to my therapies. I was determined to get the virus out of my system, or at least to learn how to keep it well and truly under control.

My confidence in the therapies was well founded. For months now I have been free of all the major symptoms for the first time since the illness started. When I think back to how ill I was, this seems an unbelievable achievement, but even now every day brings another small improvement. There are still relapses, times of weakness and tiredness, but these can be controlled and they pass quickly. Thankfully, I am once again able to work and play with the energy and enthusiasm that I believed had gone for ever.

My story of illness and diagnosis is not at all unusual. Since finding my way back to health I have met many other people who are suffering from this debilitating disease. Many of them have terrible tales to tell, not only about the physical and mental problems caused by the illness, but also about their difficulties with the medical establishment. I have met children whom the authorities wanted to label 'phobic' or 'educationally subnormal' because of their illness. If these kids had not received an accurate diagnosis in time, their lives would have been blighted still further by the stigma of having had psychiatric treatment. I do not like to think about the probable large number of children who have not received an accurate diagnosis. For them, psychiatric treatment is mistreatment.

Adults, too, are wrongly diagnosed in all sorts of painful and humiliating ways. A large number, particularly women, are told by their doctors that they are neurotic, menopausal, hysterical or emotionally unbalanced. They are then pressured into accepting anti-depressants or other psycho-active drugs, and pushed into psychiatric therapy. I cannot emphasize too strongly how damaging this can be. We can only hope that now there is more known about the disease, more local GPs will come to understand it and deal with their patients properly.

In the meantime, we must all develop a slightly wary attitude towards the medical establishment. Those of you who may think that you have the illness, and those who have just been diagnosed, should learn a vital lesson from all of us who have suffered in the past: your doctor should be your friend. By this I mean simply that your doctor should be someone whom you can relate to easily, and someone who you feel confident is on your side, is willing to be supportive and is concerned enough to help you find suitable treatment. A doctor who is ignorant about the disease, sceptical about your problems or unwilling to seek out solutions will do you more harm than good. If your doctor is unsympathetic, do not be frightened to ask for a second opinion or to be referred to a specialist. If all else fails, get in touch with one of the M.E. groups. They probably know of sufferers in your area who have already been through these problems and have found a sympathetic medic.

Having drawn attention to the problem of finding a suitable medical adviser, I must also make you aware of your responsibility towards the doctor you have found. People like myself, whose symptoms include intense mental disorientation and lack of comprehension, can create problems for doctors. It is vital that doctors get a clear picture of exactly what is happening to you. If you cannot understand the doctors' questions, cannot remember what has been happening to you or cannot speak coherently, you will not be able to give your advisers all the information about your symptoms that they need. If this happens, your doctors will be making decisions based on only a partial knowledge of your situation. Obviously, this reduces your chances of being helped, so you must find some other way to communicate effectively.

Many times in the early days of my illness I went along to the doctor's surgery or the hospital in a state of total confusion. I could not understand anything I saw or heard. I could not remember clearly. I could not speak without slurring and mumbling. In short, I was in no way able to communicate the complex range of ailments and symptoms which had taken over my life.

In my more lucid moments, I realized that this was a ridiculous waste of time for everyone concerned. I could not expect to get any help unless I could state my problems reasonably clearly. So I got into the habit of keeping a notepad lying around. On this pad I would jot down notes about my symptoms as and when they occurred. In this way I always had up-to-date information about my state of health. Just before every appointment I could read through the list to refresh my memory, or, if I was particularly ill, I could simply hand the notes to the doctor when I arrived. During the times when I was too ill to write, I would ask a friend to make the notes for me.

Keeping notes like this might seem an incredible chore when you are ill, but it is a very effective way to ensure that your doctor fully understands what is happening to you. Alternatively, if you share a house with friends or family, you could ask them to describe your situation to the doctor for you, making sure that they include even the minor symptoms. However you decide to do it, you must ensure that you communicate fully and properly with your medics. This is the only way in which you can improve your chances of prompt and correct diagnosis and support.

The importance of a correct diagnosis cannot be overstressed. All the time you are in doubt about the cause of your illness, you are fighting against an invisible enemy, never knowing how, when or where it might strike next. This leaves you in a constant state of doubt and fear. The uncertainty about what is happening to your body can be unbelievably stressful. It is all too easy to imagine that you have a brain tumour or something equally fatal when you are constantly confused and in pain. Even if you consciously know that these worries are ridiculous, at lower levels your mind remains restless and anxious. As soon as you get a positive diagnosis, your mind is put at rest and the energy tied up in worrying is freed to help you overcome the illness. For people who have been ill for a long time, finally getting a positive diagnosis produces a feeling of relief and well-being which borders on euphoria.

This is strange when you consider that a diagnosis of M.E. almost always amounts to a sentence of years of pain and difficulty. In my experience, the relief stems from the fact that the enemy has become visible. At last you know exactly what it is that you are up against. You know that the disease is not fatal, and that it is not degenerative. Knowing that you will not die from M.E., you can start devoting all of your energy to learning to live with it. And this is the first step towards conquering your illness.

Living with M.E. is a constant exercise in the fine art of self-awareness. Gradually you learn about your own tolerances and limitations: how much you can do without suffering for it later; how long you can concentrate; how late you can stay up; how early you can rise; how much you can work, or play, or write, or talk, or watch TV, or drink, or think, or listen, or walk, or read, or eat, or ... or ... or ... All of these things, which you used to take for granted, suddenly have to be measured and carefully considered. You have to remain constantly aware of your resources of strength and to take very good care that you do not exhaust them.

Of course, your limitations will be completely different from everyone else's. You will find that your tolerance for some things is much greater than for others. For example, like many patients,

I sufferered badly in the middle of the night. I would wake up with a high fever, dripping with sweat, in great pain and mental confusion. Unable to sleep again, my mind would spiral into the pain, depression would set in, and I would spend the rest of the night in utter misery, feeling too weak and sick even to cry. This happened every night for months. I desperately needed something to occupy me during those long, lonely nights. My tolerance for books, magazines and TV was absolutely nil – I could not understand a single thing – but I found that I could tolerate playing cards. Thus began a habit which has persisted until today. For some reason my mind could take in and make sense of the thousands of games of patience I played through this period, when everything else was completely beyond me.

Having discovered this, I had found a weapon to help fight off the loneliness and misery of those dark nights. I no longer felt so helpless and hopeless, which was a great step forward. Instead of fearing the nights, I knew that I could get through them with a minimum of suffering.

Of course, the next step was to exploit this tolerance for all it was worth. I asked friends to go to the library and take out books of card games, so that I had a wide range of games to suit my mental states: some demanding, others less so. I played the simple games when I was ill, and the small triumph of winning helped to keep me cheerful and optimistic. During convalescent phases, when my mind became more agile and responsive, I played the most demanding games to fend off boredom and frustration.

In playing cards I had found an occupation to help focus my mind outside myself, away from the illness. This provided valuable breathing spaces in each day when I forgot, as much as was possible, the pain and weakness which afflicted me the rest of the time. Without this, every day would have been totally dominated by illness.

Other people have found different ways of achieving these breathing spaces. One lady I know found that she could tolerate making simple flower arrangements when she was too ill for other pursuits, so she spent sleepless nights arranging and rearranging pretty decorations for her friends and her home. During periods of great mental alertness, she read books on Japanese arrangements and began to experiment with new shapes, colours and combinations. In the same way that I now always keep a pack of cards around the house, she keeps a few bunches of dried flowers in a cupboard as an insurance against those bad days and nights that crop up every now and again.

Anything which is physically undemanding and sufficiently stimulating to interest the mind will help you get into your own breathing space and away from your problems for a short while. The benefits of this cannot be overestimated. It allows you to realize that life does exist outside your illness and that you can do something competently, even if it is only playing cards against yourself. Mentally and emotionally it gives you something to hold on to, and it prevents you from losing all self-respect and all expectation of health. Most important of all, it provides a little relief from your constant awareness of a heavy, painful body and a confused, unhappy mind.

Learning about the breathing spaces was an important development in my approach to the illness, and the relief the spaces provided helped me to concentrate more fully on the therapies which were proving successful. This book is all about the breathing spaces which can be found in the therapies themselves, and is written with the aim of helping every individual sufferer find a safe, simple treatment which will provide the much needed relief.

Most of the therapies in this book are suitable for the individual to use at home, but some require the assistance of a professional practitioner. In every case, people who suffer from myalgic encephalomyelitis have found the treatment successful. The therapies explained and recommended here have all been approved by other sufferers and thus hopefully will provide you with a short list of treatments known to be effective, from which you can select the ones most suitable for your needs.

Before examining the therapies in greater detail, it is sensible to take a closer look at the illness. Making the enemy fully visible will help you to replace uncertainty with understanding of exactly what is happening inside your own body. Understanding what the disease can do will help you to defend yourself against it with more success.

2

THE DISEASE ...

Myalgic encephalomyelitis is caused by a virus – probably one of the 80 or more viruses known collectively as the 'entero' virus group which enter the body through the digestive system and which affect the brain, nerves and muscles of the sufferer. Having said that, there is very little other information available. Since the virus was discovered, an immense effort has been made by researchers to find out the full story of this elusive germ. As yet, no major breakthroughs have taken place, but gradually small pieces of the puzzle are falling into position, and there is generally a feeling of optimism that we shall soon understand the causes of this illness more fully.

M.E. has been around for a very long time. Outbreaks of varying severity have occurred all over the world and until recently no one could explain what caused the malady. In 1955 an outbreak at the Royal Free Hospital in London affected doctors and nurses, bringing the work of the hospital to a grinding halt. The Royal Free disease, as it was called, was said to have been caused by mass hysteria, which is one of those explanations which really explains nothing. None of the doctors who suggested this explanation could define what mass hysteria was, or how it worked or why it should affect doctors and nurses but not patients. None the less, mass hysteria became the official explanation for the events at the Royal Free.

An outbreak in Iceland, which affected most of the inhabitants of a small town, received much the same response. Newspapers reported the medical authorities as saying that the infamous mass hysteria was to blame for the townspeople's illness. The illness itself was unimaginatively referred to as Icelandic disease.

This ridiculous theory of mass hysteria lent some semblance of scientific credibility to the notion that M.E. sufferers were all mentally unstable. It has taken many years for the medical establishment to realize and admit that they have been seriously mistaken, and even now many doctors are unaware of the true nature of M.E. Doctors who have, in the past, developed the idea that M.E. is a psychosomatic disorder can be very reluctant to face up to the proof that the disease results from a viral infection. Some GPs still assess sufferers as malingerers or hysterics and tell them to 'pull themselves together'. Fortunately, many doctors are more understanding than this and make the effort to keep up with recent developments in research. They are willing to acknowledge that their patients are suffering from a debilitating infection and offer valuable support and advice. Hopefully, before much longer, all doctors will adopt this more sensible and sensitive approach.

In the meantime, we are left with many unanswered questions about the illness. For example, we do not know how people catch it. Although there is no firm evidence to prove the case one way or another, it seems unlikely that it is transmitted from person to person. If this is correct then the virus must exist, and possibly breed, somewhere in the environment. This, of course, would explain how large groups of people can catch it at the same time, as happened in Iceland, at the Royal Free Hospital and, more recently, at a school in Scotland where all the staff contracted the illness.

Another important question concerns the duration of the illness. Again, no firm evidence is available one way or the other, but various authorities are suggesting that it lasts for two years, five years, ten years or even indefinitely. As there is so much difference between the various estimates, none of them can be taken seriously. I suggest that you ignore all of them and concentrate on getting well in the shortest possible time.

Although it should not be long before researchers can fully explain the hows and whys of M.E., until they can we must resign ourselves to being rather in the dark about the illness. However, even without scientific evidence, much useful information can be gained by examining how people with the illness find that it affects them. Having talked to many sufferers, I have found that the general opinion is that there is a pattern to the illness which is more or less the same in most cases. Understanding this pattern helps people to know what to expect from the illness, and being forewarned in this way can prevent a lot of pain and worry.

The first sign of M.E. is usually a virus infection of some kind, quite often a form of gastric flu and sometimes with respiratory complications, that takes longer than usual to clear up, and though the symptoms of the infection gradually disappear, the patient is left with the symptoms of M.E.: extreme tiredness, fatigue, coldness, etc. Very often people assume that these are just the after-effects of the flu or whatever they had. It is only when it gets more severe and continues for weeks or months that they start to think that something else may be wrong.

This first stage of the illness is very important. Assuming that the M.E. symptoms are just the after-effects of the virus infection, many people return to a normal lifestyle and try to work through the weakness. This is a serious mistake. Forcing yourself to work, even if it is only doing minor things like dusting and shopping, can intensify all of the symptoms and prolong the illness greatly. If you really push yourself hard to get things done, it can prompt your symptoms to degenerate into a chronic state. If you have had such an infection and for any reason suspect that instead of the normal convalescent weakness you have M.E., see your doctor at once and ask for a test.

The symptoms of M.E. are not unlike normal convalescent weakness. When you are getting over flu, for example, you feel tired, weak and shaky, and simple tasks require more effort than normal. M.E. patients suffer all of these symptoms constantly and in an extreme form, but often they have muscular pain and swelling, back and head pain and extreme coldness as well. Other obvious symptoms are severe memory lapses, lack of comprehension and rapid mood swings.

In a minority of sufferers, the illness will continue exactly as it started for a lengthy period, sometimes for years. For the majority, it is a different story. The illness continues for a period of weeks or months (often not more than eight months); then the patient starts to improve. Day by day the symptoms recede and the patient starts to feel human again. This convalescent period is wonderful, but it is a time to take great care because all is not as it seems. Although you feel stronger, you are still not strong. Many sufferers, fooled by the improvement, assume that they are recovering and start to live a more strenuous life. As soon as they attempt things which are too much for them, the illness returns with speed and force.

M.E. sufferers soon learn that to give themselves the best chance of health they have to remain constantly aware of their energy levels and never tire themselves to the point where the illness can take over again. This can impose very strict limitations on your lifestyle. Some people can work only part-time, if at all. Others have to ensure that they get to bed early every night. Others must rest in the afternoon, or after exercise. It is difficult to adjust to the fact that the illness is always in the background, ready to emerge again if you give it the slightest chance. If you do not adjust to this new fact of life, you will probably suffer relapse after relapse. Fighting the illness by making an extra effort to get things done is a natural but very foolish response. Paradoxically the only way to beat the virus is to give in to it. Rest and relaxation are the only sure ways to relieve the symptoms and prevent constant attacks.

The periods of convalescence and relatively good health following bouts of illness can be extended by cautious and sensible living on the part of the sufferer. But even this does not necessarily prevent relapses. Many people have found that the illness has a cycle, so that at various times of the year they are prone to relapse no matter how careful they are. A common pattern is to relapse in autumn or winter and recover in spring.

Relapses, whether stemming from over-exertion or natural causes, tend to be as bad or worse than previous bouts every time. For many people the first bout of illness is the weakest and in each subsequent bout the illness gets stronger and takes longer to recover from. This pattern of gradual degeneration is very common, but in most cases it eventually halts of its own accord. At this point you may still have relapses but they will be no worse than the preceding ones. Unfortunately, this is often because they can get no worse – you have become as ill as you can get.

So, overall the illness seems usually to follow a pattern of bouts and remissions. The length of each can vary from person to person, and also from time to time in the same individual. Many things can trigger relapses, but in all cases mental or physical over-exertion is a major cause. When you are in a bout of illness, something as simple as making a cup of tea can amount to over-exertion, so you have to be very careful.

Although it has now been proved that M.E. is an illness with an organic cause, it seems to me and to other sufferers that there is a strong psychological component which should not be overlooked. Everyday experience shows us that our feelings have a very strong effect on everything we do. When you are in a state of sadness or depression you feel slow and heavy, and living is a constant struggle. Conversely, when you feel happy and outgoing you seem to have a constant flow of energy at your fingertips. This is a simple example of the way in which moods can colour, or even control, our physical strength and stamina. With M.E. exactly the same is true, and to a heightened degree. Whether this is because of interference produced by the virus's effect on the emotional centres of the brain, or whether it simply happens because physical weakness allows the emotional influence to become dominant, is not known. Nevertheless, it is a very real effect.

One lady I know had been in a remission period for almost a year. She had achieved this state by using alternative therapies and generally taking a sensible approach to life. She had returned to work full-time and felt that she was in control of the illness. One day, without any warning, she began to experience strong pain in her leg muscles. These muscles were where she had been affected most severely during the worst of her illness. Realizing that she had obviously done something wrong and allowed the illness to creep up on her, she tried to figure out what her mistake had been. She checked the amounts of exercise she had taken, made sure her diet had been good and thought back to discover whether she had been losing any sleep. Everything in these areas was fine, so she was at a loss to place exactly what had gone wrong.

This lady was in one of the caring services, and over the week previous to her problem she had had to deal with several cases which had upset her badly. Once she realized that it was the emotional turmoil which had triggered the leg pain, she could deal with it quickly and effectively by talking out her feelings and thus removing the emotional burden. With this internal pressure gone, she immediately felt better and has had no more pain since. This is a very important lesson for all M.E. sufferers. Your inner mental and emotional energies are just as important as the outer physical ones, and must be protected in the same way.

When you are constantly cold, tired and in pain, 'listening' to your body becomes almost second nature. You are aware of how you are feeling from moment to moment, often uncomfortably so, and immediately know when your body starts telling you that you have done enough or too much. This is almost a built-in instinct, so it is fairly simple to bring it into full conscious awareness. It is not nearly as simple to 'listen' to your feelings in the same way. Many of us go through life carrying a heavy load of unhappiness, fear, doubt, insecurity or anger of which we are hardly conscious. This load always has a bad effect on us mentally and physically, but when we are healthy the effect can easily be overlooked or ignored. When we have M.E., this load suddenly becomes intolerable. It puts a stress on our systems that we can no longer bear. It causes an immediate and dramatic worsening of all symptoms and can cause greater long-term difficulties unless it is removed. Talking to someone who is understanding and sympathetic is the best cure for these inner difficulties, but self-awareness and the inner therapies mentioned later in this book are even better because they prevent the situation of stress arising in the first place.

Just as anything that intensifies your emotions – making you feel down, uncomfortable or uptight – complicates the illness, physical stress is harmful too. Anything that gives you a sensation of tension should be strictly avoided whilst you are in bouts of illness, and only experienced to a reasonable extent when you are in convalescence or remission. Physical tension is merely the outward sign of inner stress and discomfort, so by avoiding things and situations which cause you physical tension you will be relieving the burden on your inner self too.

One of the things which I have always found stressful is travelling by public transport. I avoid buses completely and only take trains when there is no practical alternative. A journey by train leaves me feeling very uptight, particularly if I have had to travel during the rush hour. The physical tension it produces is the outward echo of an inner stress caused by the journey. I have an intense dislike of being in a small space with many other people and this feeling strongly influences me mentally and physically whenever I have to make a journey by public transport.

When I am feeling fit I can cope with the effects of this stress, but since I have had M.E. I have found that train travel will wipe out all my resources for the rest of the day. I soon came to realize that I had a simple choice. I could either waste my mental and physical energy on a stressful pursuit, leaving myself drained and prone to illness, or I could use my resources to feel well and happy and to achieve something worthwhile. It was not difficult to decide between the two. I have adjusted my lifestyle to eliminate this stressful activity to the greatest possible degree.

Unfortunately, having M.E. is not a simple business. It is not a case of being ill, getting well and then carrying on life as before. If you wish to reduce the illness to manageable proportions and make the best use of your time and energy, you are forced to make changes. Some of these changes are simple, outward ones: altering your routine, regularly using alternative therapies, allowing for your illness where you cannot work round it. Other changes are more complex, to do with your inner world. Learning to 'listen' to your emotions is the first and most important of these, and this can lead you to change your attitudes, beliefs and expectations.

One sufferer I knew, when talking about the illness, said, 'It's been awful, but in a way it has been good too. I have found out so much about myself that I never knew before. I am more capable of living a happy life now than I ever was before I fell ill.' I think that this is a wonderful attitude and agree with it wholeheartedly. Even though you set out to make your life better by understanding the disease, you end up making a happier life for yourself by understanding yourself in a way you never have before. Along the way you can lose all sorts of negative feelings and gain a full knowledge of what is important to you. When you regain your health you may find that you have a new and positive attitude to many things in your life.

Having examined the overall pattern of illness that you may expect, let's now look more closely at the day-to-day effect of the virus on your body – the symptoms.

3

... AND ITS SYMPTOMS

Part of the reason why M.E. was thought to be a psychosomatic disorder for so long is that different sufferers reported different symptoms. One might complain of coldness and headaches, while another sought help for fevers and pain in the limbs. Until the virus was identified, there was little logical reason to assume that these two people were suffering from the same disease. However, what was overlooked for a long time was the fact that only the major symptoms were being taken into account when a diagnosis was attempted. Once the minor symptoms were also considered, a pattern emerged which linked almost all M.E. sufferers.

M.E. can produce a vast range of symptoms, affecting all parts of the body. In a few people, one symptom will be dominant and the others absent or slight enough to cause no concern. In the vast majority of cases, there will be a group of dominant symptoms complicated by minor problems of many different types. By noting all of the symptoms, major and minor, you develop a list of symptoms which are familiar to all sufferers. The only difference between individuals is the severity of each symptom. This is why people can sometimes seem to be suffering from completely different diseases. In fact, it is the same disease, with the emphasis slightly altered in each case. Every sufferer experiences an unique combination of the various symptoms, but they are the same symptoms in every case.

This difference in symptoms complicates the whole matter of treatment. As there is no overall cure, therapists can only hope to treat individual symptoms successfully as and when they arise. This means that the therapy which works for one sufferer may have little or no effect on another. Also, because the minor symptoms can change from day to day, or even from hour to hour, it is very difficult to develop a course of treatment which is constantly effective. It is necessary always to keep a weather-eye on your symptoms and stay alert to the changes which occur. In this way you will always know which of the symptoms are your major priority for treatment and, hopefully, for relief. Use the following list to help you decide which problems are your priorities and concentrate on finding suitable treatment for these first. Once you have achieved some relief, then you can experiment to find successful ways of dealing with the minor symptoms.

If you have just been diagnosed, some of the symptoms in the following list may be new to you. Do not worry about this. Not every sufferer experiences every symptom. Your pattern of illness is probably already established, so if you have not had a particular symptom already, you may not get it at all. Your major symptoms will only change slowly, if they change at all, and the list can help you expect and adapt to the changes of minor symptoms that all of us who have M.E. experience.

Those of you who are wondering whether you have M.E. should use the following list as a guide-line. If you have experienced several or many of the symptoms over a lengthy period, then contact your doctor to ask his advice or request a blood test for a positive diagnosis. If you have had severe trouble with one or more symptoms, a visit to your doctor is also indicated. Do not forget that there are other causes for all of the individual symptoms on the list, and many of these other causes are far easier to cure than M.E. Even if you should eventually receive a confirmed diagnosis of M.E., do not be disheartened. The sooner you find out, the sooner you can learn to live with the illness and find an effective remedy.

The symptoms

Tiredness

I have put this symptom first because I have found that it is perhaps the most widespread of all amongst sufferers. Very few are lucky enough to escape problems in this area. Like all of the symptoms, it can vary enormously in its severity, so I shall try to illustrate the full spectrum of its influence.

Tiredness was one of my own first symptoms, and has been one of the longest lasting. In its strongest form, it can totally disrupt your lifestyle because in every waking moment you have an intense yearning to sleep. When sitting or lying down, there is no way in which you can stop your eyes closing. When moving around, your only thought is of a chair or bed. You constantly feel as though you have been up all night at a particularly energetic party. Even though you sleep as much as sixteen hours a day, you wake up feeling totally unrefreshed and want to go straight back to bed.

In a milder form, the fatigue is like the after-effects of flu. You feel relatively strong first thing in the morning, but by the afternoon your strength is at its end. Afternoon naps and early nights are very appealing, and are also a very sensible way to treat this symptom. You feel slightly below par most of the time, as though you had not had quite enough sleep the previous night. Even so, you will probably find yourself sleeping much more than normal.

At best, the tiredness becomes a minor inconvenience. You may have to buy a louder alarm clock to make sure that you get up in the morning, and you will probably find that by mid- to late afternoon you are feeling low. I always have a low period between 4 and 6 p.m. To allow for this, I always make sure that nothing too energetic or demanding is scheduled for this period when I am at my weakest. By early evening I have picked up again and feel reasonably alert until bedtime, which I make sure is at a reasonable hour. This pattern of highs and lows is very common in periods of convalescence and remission.

During the worst stages of fatigue there is little that you can do to help yourself except give in to the demand for sleep and more sleep. Some sufferers report that stimulants prescribed by the doctor can help, but the majority find that they should be avoided. In its mildest form, the best treatment for fatigue is to use self-awareness and will-power: be aware of your low periods during the day and work around them, establishing a regular routine that you can make yourself keep to. The mid-way form will respond well to the various treatments outlined later.

Weakness

This is also a very widespread symptom and it is most often experienced together with tiredness.

Muscular weakness is one of the most frustrating symptoms. Even if you are feeling otherwise all right, the weakness can prevent you from doing anything. When it is at its worst, simple actions like standing, sitting and lifting light objects become extremely difficult, and walking can be wellnigh impossible. Sufferers may have to be confined to bed or a wheelchair during chronic phases.

Usually the weakness is not as severe as this. Nonetheless, it is still a definite handicap. In the more common milder form, the lack of physical strength makes life difficult in any number of small ways. Making a cup of tea seems to require the effort more often associated with climbing Everest. Bottles and jars have to be opened by a helpful friend. Taps cannot be turned on and off, heavy pots and pans cannot be used and even heavy clothing can sometimes present problems. Anything requiring muscular effort becomes immensely difficult. At this stage sufferers should beware of exercise of any sort. Frustration can make you attempt to do things which are too strenuous. The result will often be a relapse into greater weakness, and if too much exercise is taken it can provoke the symptom into becoming chronic.

As with the tiredness, the mildest form of weakness is simply a scaled-down version of the intense symptom. You feel that your muscles do not have the strength and resilience that they should have. Like tiredness, this symptom is best treated with self-awareness and will-power. Arrange your days so that the more strenuous activities are attempted when you are at your brightest, and do as little as possible during your low periods. Once you have established a good routine, stick to it with every ounce of will-power you possess. Do not be tempted to do the spring-cleaning or go out with friends when you know you should be resting.

Many people have found that muscle weakness is a very sensitive symptom to deal with. It gives you a very clear indication of your current reserves of strength, but if you overstep your limitations at all you will suffer for it in the days or weeks to come. Weakness is best treated with any of the relaxation-based therapies, but acupuncture, acupressure, reflexology and hypnotism have all been suggested as effective therapies. On a preventive basis, you should make every effort to ensure that your diet includes plenty of energy-giving foods.

Pain

The bad news is that this illness can cause intense pain in any part of the body. The good news is that no sufferers seem to have pain all over, all of the time. You will probably find that you usually have difficulties in one particular area and are free of pain elsewhere.

The most common pain is in the head, neck and/or back. It is very similar to a migraine headache: continuous sharp bursts which seem to echo round your skull and down your spine. This is often accompanied by extreme light sensitivity and nausea. Unfortunately, there is little that can be done to help, and the headaches can continue for long periods. Relaxation is the therapy which brings most relief in the long term, and pain-killers should be used when necessary to provide short-term relief. It is worthwhile to try different kinds of pain-killers. I have found that some brands are more suited to me than others, and these are much more effective. Those containing Ibuprofen are the ones which help me most, and when I recommend these brands to other sufferers they are usually pleased by their effectiveness.

As well as having the migraine-type headaches, you may well find that you become more prone to the normal sort. These centre particularly around the eyes and thump away endlessly. Sometimes they fade away into the background and disappear, but often the only thing which will stop them is a good night's sleep.

Muscular pain is very common and it is not always associated with the other muscular problems. At worst the muscles grow extremely sensitive to pressure and the lightest touch can be extremely painful. This happens particularly in the long muscles of the arms and legs. They can also feel hard to the touch, and quite severe swelling can develop. In this case, avoid all exercise if possible. In its weaker form, muscular pain is a continuous dull ache which escalates to a burning sensation if you exercise too much.

Nerve pain is usually very mild – a tingling, twitching or irritated sensation just below the surface of the skin. Occasionally people complain of this escalating to a neuralgia-type pain, but this is relatively uncommon.

Joint and bone pain is extremely hard to describe. When you have it, you feel as though your bones are sore and tired – worn out, in fact. I have never come across a severe case of this type of pain, but it is frequently an unpleasant undercurrent to all the other symptoms. It usually centres in the spine, arms or hands.

Chest pain is one of the most frightening symptoms. Many sufferers have thought that they were going into a heart attack when this problem has struck. The pain comes in stabs and bursts and seems to centre around the heart. It can be accompanied by palpitations or missed heartbeats. The pain is very much aggravated by quick breathing or by rapid chest movements such as happen when you laugh, and it can be triggered by either. The pain will pass quickly if you sit quietly, relax and breathe slowly and deeply for a few minutes. Obviously, if you have any history of heart problems or are in a high-risk group, you should check with your doctor immediately if you have problems in this area.

Tremors

People who have not suffered from this symptom seem to consider it a minor thing, but in practice it is an embarrassing and awkward problem. The muscles of the arms and legs, particularly the hands and feet, twitch continuously, so that there is a constant shaking and quivering of the affected part of the body. It is not painful, but if the major muscles of the arms or legs are affected it can prevent you from walking properly or carrying anything. Even if only the extremities are shaking it is highly irritating if it continues over a lengthy period. It also makes you seem very clumsy because you keep spilling drinks or tripping over your own feet. The relaxation-based therapies, biochemic remedies and homoeopathy can all help with this symptom.

Temperature

There are many temperature abnormalities, but by far the most common is coldness. This can take the form of cold hands and feet or a general all-over chilliness, or it can vary according to your other symptoms – the more your muscles ache, the colder you become, for example. At its worst it becomes very intense, and the sufferer will be shivering no matter how high the central heating is set or how many warm clothes are worn. At this level, the coldness is always accompanied by a worsening of all other symptoms, and perhaps it is caused by this worsening. There is no escaping it, but long hot baths can relieve the situation for reasonable periods. Most sufferers find that their temperature is constantly below normal, by a degree or more, even when they are feeling relatively healthy.

Sudden increases in temperature can also occur after any exertion and they usually occur following food. If you take small amounts of food fairly often, this can help you to maintain a reasonable body temperature.

Fevers

Sometimes intense fevers can occur when the illness is at its worst, and I certainly suffered from them, but more often they are low grade fevers with body temperature rising to no more than 100°F/38°C. My fevers usually struck at night, and if you happen to be awake when one starts you can feel your temperature rising minute by minute. If you are asleep during the onset, as is usually the case, the first thing you become aware of as you are woken by the extreme heat is sweat – and plenty of it. At the very least you will be damp and sticky when you wake, and very often the sweat is so heavy that the bed has to be changed before you get back into it.

These night sweats can be ferocious. I have been through several long periods of them, waking up two or three times every night with sweat running off me. After towelling off and changing the bed, I would fall asleep quickly, only to wake up an hour later wringing wet again. The whole thing was physically exhausting and emotional demoralizing.

After one particularly awful day, when I did not have the

energy to go and get myself any food or drink, I fell into bed early and went into the usual sequence of night sweats. After the first one I climbed back into bed, anxious for sleep and lay there wide awake. This was confusing because I normally fell straight back to sleep as soon as I was cool and dry. Then my temperature started to go up. Soon my mind was affected by the fever and I grew increasingly hazy and delirious as my temperature climbed. I laid there for what seemed like a month, growing hotter and hotter. Then I realized that I was not sweating, and everything fell into place. I was dehydrated, and without the sweat evaporating to cool me there was nothing to control my temperature. I forced myself out of bed to go and get a glass of water, and within minutes of drinking it I was sweating again and cooling off rapidly.

This provided a valuable lesson. If you experience the fevers and night sweats, make sure that you increase your intake of liquids to compensate for all the water lost through sweating. To dehydrate in a fever is very dangerous and can damage you permanently. Also, every time you sweat heavily you are losing salt and other important nutrients from the body, so it is probably wise to ensure that your diet is more than adequate during these periods.

Experience taught me that pain-killers are very useful in small amounts to break the fever and bring your temperature down. If you are going through a bad period and can expect a disturbed night, then half or a quarter of a tablet before bedtime will help to ensure a good night's rest. If an unexpected fever wakes you up, take the same dose and it will prevent further disturbances.

Sleep patterns and disturbances

Night sweats and fevers, as described above, are the most noticeable of the sleep disturbances which occur with this disease. The others are much less worrying, but can still be a little disturbing. For those of us, like myself, who rarely remember their dreams, the Panavision, Technicolor epics which the illness sometimes produces can be quite shocking. Waking up with your head ringing to the sights and sounds of this unexpected dreamscape can be alarming at first. Learn to relax and enjoy this built-in entertainment system. Think of it as a compensation for all of the difficult times.

Apart from sweats and dreams, you could find yourself waking up in the middle of the night for any number of reasons – for a drink or a snack or to go to the toilet. Then there are times when there is no good reason to wake up; you simply do. Whether or not you feel hungry or thirsty, you will often find that some food or a hot drink will send you back to sleep quickly and safely. Always avoid sleeping-tablets unless there really is no other option.

Disturbances of your sleep patterns are always unpleasant. When they are frequent it is like living with permanent jet-lag. Every body has its own rhythms, its own preferences for when to sleep and when to wake. Many sufferers find that their illness throws their sleep patterns into total disarray, and they have continually to adjust their lifestyles to cope with irregular sleep needs.

Sufferers usually find that they require more sleep than normal, but instead of taking it in one single block at night, their bodies tell them to rest at various points during the day. As I have already said, I have a daily 'low' between 4 and 6 p.m. At that time I feel tired and drained and would like nothing better than to lie down. When I was really ill I had to sleep then. If I had deliberately kept myself awake (if that were possible), it would have weakened me and perhaps triggered a relapse. During the bad periods of illness you need all the sleep you can get, to allow your mind and body to replenish themselves. Once you achieve a convalescent state, or even remission, you can retrain your mind and body to sleep once in every twenty-four hours.

Make up your mind to accept the fact that while you are ill you will feel the need to sleep at odd times of the day. As long as this does not interfere too much with your sleep at night, give in to it. As you start to get better you can rest instead of sleeping during the day, and this will gradually alter your sleep pattern to a more suitable rhythm.

Sweats

Some sufferers have the unpleasant experience of sweats which are apparently unconnected with temperature changes. These sweats can happen at any time, but are usually day-time events rather than night-time ones. The sweats are unusual in that only one part of the body might be affected. For example, the thighs, lower legs, arms, armpits, neck and back can all be affected individually. No anti-perspirant will prevent these sweats, and no deodorant can mask the odour, which is sometimes awful.

Feeling just one part of your body sweating is a very peculiar sensation, and as yet no one knows how or why these localized sweats are caused. However, there is reason to believe that they are healthy. Any sweat contains wastes and toxins that the body wants to throw off. Heavy or badly smelling sweats are likely to be a simple defence mechanism which allows the body to free itself of all sorts of rubbish that have accumulated in your system. Unfortunately, it is these wastes which produce the awful smell, which can be highly embarrassing for hygiene and odour-conscious sufferers. Console yourself with the fact that your body is protecting itself by sweating out wastes in this way, and try the treatment described under hydrotherapy to alleviate this irritating symptom. You will find that regularly using a therapy which causes you to sweat can prevent both these localized sweats and the more wearing night sweats.

Secondary infections

M.E. is a constant attack on your body's natural defences. Over a period of time, your defences become worn down to the point where you are more susceptible to other infections than you would normally be. Your immune system, which normally fights off invading germs, becomes depresssed and can no longer react as quickly or effectively as it should. This allows other infections, called secondary infections, to take hold. Once established they can be very difficult to get rid of.

Some people experience this immune depression as a tendency to catch colds, flu and other bugs more often, and find that once caught they can last for several weeks at a time. Others find that they persistently get infections in the same places. My throat was a definite weak spot in this regard, and I also regularly suffered from urethritis.

Usually the secondary infections are relatively minor. A healthy person could overcome them within a few days. However, because of the depressed state of your immune system, minor infections can become a major problem.

To take the common cold as an example, a healthy person usually overcomes the virus within a week. For an M.E. sufferer, it could take three or four weeks. And the story does not end there. Any secondary infection can stress your system beyond its ability to cope, and all of your M.E. symptoms can return or intensify with great speed and force.

The only truly effective way to treat secondary infections is not to catch them in the first place. In this case prevention is certainly better, and easier, than cure. You cannot defend yourself completely against all of the many different bugs that people are prone to, but you should at least take elementary precautions. Do not visit friends and relatives who have coughs, colds, flu or any other catchable disease, and do not allow these people to visit you.

If one part of your body is particularly susceptible to infections, protect it from every sort of preventable stress. For instance, with my throat always poised on the brink of infection I quickly learnt that to give it the best chance of health I had to cut out all of the things that might irritate it. I cut alcohol and other strong drinks out of my diet, along with hot and spicy foods. Then, the unkindest cut of all, I had to cut out as much talking as possible. These measures allowed my throat to recuperate, and gave it a better chance of fighting off any new potential infections. This, in turn, helped my general health. With no recurrent throat problems my system was that much more able to fight off the primary infection – M.E.

Candida and thrush

A yeast-like fungal micro-organism known as *Candida albicans* lives quite naturally and, under normal circumstances, harmlessly in certain regions of the intestinal tract. It is only when the internal 'climate' of our bodies changes, allowing *Candida* to breed freely, that it causes problems in the gut, with associated infections such as thrush. Amongst the things that are known to provoke *Candida* overgrowth are an excess of sugar in the diet, overuse of antibiotics, and the contraceptive pill.

The result of *Candida* overgrowth in the gut is a depletion of the body's natural immune response system which in turn leads to a number of symptoms, including fatigue. It is a predisposing factor in M.E., and many sufferers have *Candida* problems with the related conditions of developing allergies, chronic diarrhoea or constipation, oral or vaginal thrush, amongst other symptoms.

The drug Nystatin, an anti-fungal agent, has proved useful in controlling *Candida* overgrowth, but it is not the complete answer, and the necessary strategy is one which helps the body back to health so that the gut yeasts can be naturally held in check. You should eliminate as much sugar as possible from your diet and avoid yeast-containing foods. Capricin (or caprystatin) is another anti-fungal agent which can be obtained without prescription. (BioCare, 20-24 High Street, Solihull, West Midlands, B91 3TB).

Another excellent treatment for *Candida* problems, and one which is entirely natural, is a regular dose of bacteria called acidophilus. This can be bought in most health food stores in hard capsule form and, like *Candida*, it is a normal inhabitant of our internal world. In healthy people *Candida* and acidophilus compete within the digestive tract, and this is one of the factors which prevents *Candida* getting out of control.

A regular dose of the harmless acidophilus bacteria can ensure that *Candida* does not get the chance to breed freely within us, thus preventing the *Candida*-related symptoms so many M.E. sufferers are predisposed to. Acidophilus tablets should be taken last thing at night, and chewed thoroughly before swallowing. They taste fairly pleasant, so this is no real hardship, and they can be a very effective treatment for all *Candida* problems, and as a preventative measure thereafter.

Allergies

We all have mild allergies to something in the environment, but when we are well these can be easily overlooked. If your body is weakened by illness, though, it can no longer deal with such potential allergies and they can come out with some force. Indeed, they are a major problem for long-term sufferers of M.E., and there is the connection here with *Candida* overgrowth in the gut referred to above.

Clearly you need to identify and avoid the foods which you develop allergic reactions to, but if you have severe problems you should see your doctor, or seek the advice of a qualified clinical ecologist.

Digestive disorders

Digestive disorders come in such a large variety that it is pointless to try to describe them all. However, one should definitely be noted: constipation. This is a common symptom which, for some reason, can complicate all the other symptoms enormously. Even when the constipation is mild it can, quite literally, make all your other symptoms feel ten times worse than they really are. Therefore, regular bowel movements should be of prime importance to you. Obviously it is best to prevent difficulties in this area arising by including lots of fibre in your diet. If you should have problems, it is probably best to treat yourself with a gentle natural laxative and make as many diet improvements as you can.

Debilitation

In the dictionary debilitation is defined as 'feebleness', and that is exactly how it feels. I doubt whether this is a distinct symptom of M.E. It is more likely that a combination of other symptoms – coldness, tiredness, weakness, lack of concentration, etc. – produces the feeling of being absolutely feeble. The best way to describe this state is that those in it have a total lack of stamina, mental and physical. If you think that debilitation describes your situation accurately, try to pin-point the combination of other symptoms which are active in your case, and treat these instead of the overall feebleness. Treating the root cause of the problem in this way will produce the best results.

Miscellaneous

There is a group of symptoms which are not in themselves major problems, but which can produce difficulties and worry if the sufferer is not prepared for them. Very often these symptoms can be the first to appear, and thus act as an early warning system, alerting you to the fact that unless you take care of yourself you may relapse into another bout of illness.

Pallor and M.E. throat are two classic early warning signs. 'Pallor' simply means 'paleness' and it is recognized medically as a sign of the illness. In practical terms it means that the sufferer goes white. This happens at any time up to several hours before the beginning of an attack or the worsening of symptoms. It also happens when the sufferer gets overtired or is in danger of exhausting themself. It is an infallible indicator of your state of health and should always be taken as a warning. Unfortunately, the sufferer is rarely aware of this paleness and has to rely on other people to point it out.

M.E. throat is not, as far as I know, recognized medically, but you should learn to look out for it. It is a slightly gruff quality in the voice, caused by a thickening of your saliva. It most resembles a mild attack of catarrh – your throat constantly feels a little bit clogged up. If you do not clear your throat regularly your voice tends to be rough and unreliable. Your saliva becomes noticeably thicker than usual and may well get creamy in texture and taste. This is particularly obvious after a drink of cold water. M.E. throat can last for days, weeks or months at a time, and always indicates that you are in a weakened state.

Nausea is another good warning sign for those who suffer from it. Nauseous attacks at night or early in the morning, sometimes leading to vomiting, often foreshadow an increase in problems. The other pattern of nausea, attacks lasting only minutes at any time of day, is not such a good indicator as these attacks can happen during any period of the illness.

Problems with urine retention tend to happen towards the end of a bout of illness. Having to go to the toilet frequently (and when you have to go, you really have to go), can be embarrassing and awkward. However, it is a good indicator of your convalescence. As long as the symptom persists you should remember that you should be taking things relatively easy.

Appetite disorders come in various forms at different times during the illness. During the worst of the bouts, you may find that the sight, or even the thought, of food is enough to make you sick. Alternatively, you could be permanently ravenous. If you went off food during the illness, you will probably find that in convalescence you will have sudden, sharp pangs of hunger. Within minutes you can go from feeling comfortably full to feeling as though you had been months without food. The sensation can amount almost to panic. Always give in to these hungers and get some food into your body as soon as possible. Otherwise your strength will quickly drain away, leaving you feeling weak and ill. Many people carry around some biscuits, an apple or a chocolate bar, just in case one of these starvation attacks occurs. This is a very sensible idea.

Photophobia is the technical term for light sensitivity, which is a very common problem with M.E. patients. Sound sensitivity is also common. Both of these symptoms are particularly associated with the migraine-type headaches, but they are also experienced separately. In these conditions bright light or loud sounds cause pain in the eyes and head, or ears and head respectively. Some people, like myself, find that they have no problems with artificial light but sunlight is painful. Others find that direct light of any sort causes no difficulty, but sunlight through windows is unbearable. There is very little which can be done for these conditions, but you will find that as your health improves they will gradually disappear. In the meantime, you would be well advised to invest in a pair of sunglasses, and also in some earplugs if your environment is a noisy one.

Many people find that their glands are another infallible sign of approaching illness. The glands affected are usually those in the throat but those in the armpits or groin can also react. When these glands become hard, swollen or painful you are being told in no uncertain terms to take care of yourself, as your system is weakened. Incidentally, this problem is the reason why M.E. is so often wrongly diagnosed as glandular fever.

Having examined the physical problems of M.E., now let's take a look at the other end of the spectrum – the mental and emotional symptoms. We know so little about the mind that any description of its workings, in health or illness, can only be approximate. Take the following descriptions as signposts only. Your mental and emotional experience of M.E. will be like your mind: totally unique.

Depression

Usually we use the word 'depression' to cover a mixture of feelings, such as boredom, frustration, lack of motivation and general lack of fulfilment. This is an adequate definition in day-to-day life, but real depression is something else again: the knowledge that you can never do a single thing to help yourself, can never make a constructive move and can never expect things to improve. In this state you know, beyond a shadow of a doubt, that things can only get worse. You feel trapped in a web of circumstance which cannot be cut. Nothing offers any hope, and only oblivion can release you from the continual torment of living. This true depression is a crippling illness.

M.E. causes depression by affecting the part of the brain which helps to control our emotional states. The degree of depression felt varies from person to person, and from day to day, but even the happiest of people can find themselves cast into the depths of despair. Many sufferers can tell you of the suicidal thoughts and feelings which the depression causes. Because it often strikes when all the physical symptoms are at their worst, the world, including your own body, can indeed seem a hopeless and helpless and loveless place.

The depression can drop over you within minutes, like a cloud moving over the sun. Happily, it can lift just as quickly and unexpectedly, leaving you feeling as if you have been hit by an invisible truck and miraculously escaped unhurt.

The key to dealing with all depressions, whether of the everyday or the despairing variety, is to keep one fact in mind: you will get over it. Common sense and past experience tell you that within a day or a week or a month, you will be looking back at the down time and wondering what it was all about. If you can maintain even the slightest optimism and belief in yourself, you will win through more quickly.

Most of the depression states encountered with M.E. can be overcome with the advice offered above. However, if you should find yourself in a very bad depression, and it continues beyond your ability to cope, do not hesitate to seek help from your doctor. Anti-depressant drugs are the only sensible treatment for this phase of the illness. By this I don't mean tranquillizers. Unlike tranquillizers, anti-depressants need to be taken daily for a number of weeks before they become effective in relieving symptoms. In some cases they can literally be a 'life saver', but great care must be taken because it is easy to overdose, there are side-effects, and habituation can occur.

If you are at all unsure about whether the prescribed drug is doing you good, go straight back to your doctor. Finally, be determined to use anti-depressants for as little as effectively possible, not just to lessen the chance of side-effects and possible addiction, but also because it is much healthier for you to believe in your own ability to beat the illness than to rely on drugs. Using anti-depressants is no bad thing when you need them, but the relief they provide should be used to strengthen your resolve to find a less harmful therapy which will help you to maintain your optimism.

Memory

Almost everyone I have spoken to has mentioned memory lapses as one of the most frustrating aspects of this illness. During bouts of illness, the amnesia can become extensive. Hardly any information is retained in either the short-term or the long-term memory, so making notes has to become a way of life. During convalescent periods, memory returns to a certain extent, but there are still lapses. Names, faces, telephone numbers and all sorts of other information disappear from your mind completely, or become so vague and misty that the memory is untrustworthy. Coping with this can be embarrassing and amusing by turns. Forgetting to buy an important present, or to make an important phone call, can be extremely unfortunate, and not only for yourself. On the other hand, forgetting an old friend's name can easily be turned into a joke if they understand your situation. People are usually very understanding about such things and are prepared to join in the fun if you treat the problem lightheartedly.

I well remember a three-way conversation I had with two other sufferers, Sue and Les. We all knew each other's names well, but continually lapsed. On pain of death I could not recall their proper names, but persisted in calling them Laura and Mike. Les forgot Sue's name totally, and called me Paul. Sue called me Mike, but remembered Les accurately. What was supposed to be a serious interview became quietly hysterical and we ended up giving each other rounds of applause whenever we hit on the right name.

It really is no good at all trying to force your memory into some sort of co-operation. The stress will simply aggravate your illness and cause more lapses than ever. There are indications that as the illness recedes our memories will return to something approaching normality. In the meantime, learn to make notes of all the important things and laugh off the rest as best you can.

Comprehension

Comprehension is the ability to understand the things you see or hear, the ability to make sense of information. M.E. can produce a devastating lack of comprehension. The simplest things become quite beyond your understanding. Once, during a medical examination, a doctor asked me to stand up. I did not have the foggiest idea what he meant. It was just a meaningless noise. When understanding finally dawned, I felt ashamed of my own stupidity.

This lack of comprehension can be very severe at times, as in the example I have just given. It can encompass sight, sound, touch, taste and smell. In the worst cases the person can hardly understand anything and lives as if isolated from the rest of the world. Nothing can reach across the barrier of incomprehension.

Usually the problem does not get this severe, but it does present difficulties to most sufferers. Books, TV, magazines and even conversation all become quite pointless because they are totally confusing. There is little that will dramatically improve this specific problem except improving the general state of your health, but several therapies can be helpful. Autogenics, Bach flower remedies, and royal jelly can be effective in this area, and healing is probably the most successful of all for most of the mental and emotional symptoms.

In convalescence you will probably find the lack of comprehension continuing in mild forms, getting noticeably worse when you are tired. I found that the things I heard were the first to regain their meaning, followed slowly and incompletely by visual comprehension. Even now, I still have difficulty with the written word. My spelling used to be excellent, but now I am mildly dyslexic. I cannot recognize when a word is spelt incorrectly without a massive exertion of will. No doubt the manuscript of this book was full of petty mistakes – my thanks to the editor who must have worked hard to clean it up for publication.

Concentration, or rather the lack of it, also deserves a mention here. Many people find that their ability to concentrate, to focus their mind, is badly impaired by M.E. During the worst stages of the illness it becomes difficult to concentrate on anything for more than a few minutes, or even seconds, at a time. Personally, I have no doubt that forcing your mind to concentrate is harmful during these periods. I often found that the effort of concentration needed to make an important phone call or answer a letter left me very weak and ill. There seems to be very little difference between body and mind in this respect. If you push your body beyond the limits of its strength, you will suffer for it in the following days. The same is true of your mind. In convalescence you need to push your body a little further each day to build up your strength, always being sure not to over-extend yourself. Again, the same is true of your mind. Gradually exercise your mental muscles in the same way that you exercise your physical ones. Little by little the strength will return to both.

Co-ordination and balance

Lack of co-ordination is one of the more trying symptoms for the sufferer, because it can result in what appears to be dreadful clumsiness. One lady who was particularly severely affected in this regard described herself as 'a mobile accident zone'.

The appearance of clumsiness is caused by the fact that the sufferer is no longer fully aware of exactly where their hands and feet are. Most people can reach for a cup, for example, and know almost by instinct when their hand is in the right position to pick it up safely. When co-ordination is impaired, this instinct can lead you astray. You feel as though your hand is safely positioned, but in fact it can be inches away from the object you are trying to grasp. The result of this is an endless succession of dropped or knocked over cups, plates, vases, trays and anything else that comes to hand (or, indeed, foot). At the other extremity, wrongly co-ordinated feet produce trips, stumbles and falls of every kind.

Co-ordination problems are often accompanied by, and aggravated by, a lack of balance. Sometimes this takes the form of dizziness or vertigo, but more often it is simply an inability to stand or walk straight. Walking down a perfectly straight, perfectly level corridor, I used to reel from wall to wall as though the floor beneath my feet were a wildly tossing ship. Getting into the right position to enter a door without damaging it or myself became quite a problem. It occurred to me that the doctors had overlooked one obvious symptom of M.E. – shoulders bruised from constant impact with walls and door frames.

If you have difficulty with co-ordination or balance, you must learn to take things more carefully. Realize that your body is temporarily unable to be accurate about positioning itself, and compensate by taking a little more time and effort over moving. This may not save some of your favourite china from grief, but it should reduce the wear and tear on your shoulders.

Emotional problems

Underneath this heading, I should like to mention two problems which can be as difficult for the sufferer's friends and family as they are for the sufferer. The first one is mood swings.

Mood swings affect everybody all of the time. We all go through life feeling up one minute and down the next. Very often these changes can be triggered by seemingly unimportant things, but the effects colour our whole outlook for as long as the mood lasts. With M.E. sufferers, the mood swings can be very violent and very fast. Euphoric highs followed within minutes by plummeting lows are perhaps the most severe example of this symptom.

In the high state the sufferers feel on top of the world, happy and carefree. They give off a glow of good humour and laugh at anything or nothing at all. In the low state tears take the place of laughter and the carefree feeling becomes despondency. This is often when a depression will set in.

The case I have described is a severe one, but even in the far more common milder forms the people around you will be confused and perhaps a little frightened by your rapid changes of mood. The best possible thing you can do is to tell them exactly what is going on inside you. Once they understand that your mood swings are not their fault, they can stop worrying and start to help. This also relieves you of the guilt you may start to feel for exposing your friends and family to such emotional turmoil.

The second emotional problem which you should be aware of is a possible tendency to go through anti-social phases. It can be quite distressing to have a good friend come to see you, and no sooner have they arrived than you cannot wait to see them go. The problem is even greater if it is members of your own household that you cannot bear to have around.

The reason for these anti-social phases is not yet known. Obviously at least part of it is that you are feeling weak and tired and are perhaps in pain and confusion. It is natural at these times to want to seclude yourself. However, the irregular suddenness and intensity of these feelings leads me to think that they are a true by-product, a true symptom, of the illness.

Whatever the cause of these feelings, the cure is simple. Talk about them. Take the trouble to explain to your nearest and dearest that you are going through periods when you just have to be on your own. Once they understand that this is no reflection on your relationship with them, but simply a part of your illness, they will be happy to let you have solitude when you need it and welcome you back when you are ready to communicate again.

This, then, is our list of symptoms. Let me stress again the fact that just because they are on the list it does not mean that every person who catches M.E. will suffer from them. Nobody will suffer from all of them. You will probably find that some will be with you fairly frequently, and some of the others may come and go at various times. Having read the list, you have been forewarned and forearmed. You know exactly what to expect, and need not spend precious time and energy worrying about what is happening to your body. You can, instead, focus all of your attention on combating your symptoms with the various therapies explained in the next chapter.

4

THE TREATMENT

When considering moving away from orthodox medical care
and into alternative medicine, most often people ask, 'Will it
work for me?' Unfortunately, this question cannot be answered
with a simple 'Yes' or 'No'. The only real answer is 'Yes, if you
find the right therapy.' This leads people to believe that alternative
therapies are erratic, that their results will vary from person to
person. It must be admitted that this is true, but exactly the
same must be said for orthodox treatments. The drugs
prescribed by your doctor will work for one person but not for
another. The fact that they often do work well is a testament
to the skill of the doctor in choosing the right treatment for the
right patient. An equally skilled alternative therapist will have
the same degree of success.

It is foolish to fall into the trap of thinking only in terms of
one type of medicine. Orthodox and alternative therapies are
not mutually exclusive. They can work happily together, each
bringing about benefits to the patient. Remember, however, to
keep everybody informed of your treatments. If your
homoeopath, for example, puts you on a course of tablets at
the same time as your doctor does, then make sure that they
both know what the other has prescribed. There is almost no
chance of the two treatments reacting badly together, but
orthodox drugs can sometimes inhibit the action of natural
treatments and vice versa.

Alternative therapies spring from an entirely different
understanding of health from orthodox medicine. Traditional
medical practitioners tend to think of the body as a machine,
and they will treat the parts of the machine that are not working

smoothly. In this sense, they treat the disease and not the patient. Alternative practitioners are more likely to think of the patient as a whole unit (hence the term 'holistic medicine') composed of mind and body; they believe that both these aspects of self must be treated to cure any problem. They often consider that illness is merely the outward physical reflection of an internal (mental, emotional or spiritual) problem. Therefore they work to cure the ailment by treating the problem at its roots in the patient's inner self. Bear this attitude in mind when you are considering alternative therapies and they may not seem quite so illogical or other worldly.

Another noticeable difference between orthodox medicine and alternative medicine is the speed at which the treatments work. We are all conditioned to the fact that tablets from the doctor work very speedily, usually within days if not hours. Natural preparations often work much more slowly, gently easing their way into your system and correcting imbalances. Of course, speedy cures can and do happen with natural remedies, but be prepared for the fact that you may have to be a patient patient and allow extra time for this natural magic to work.

When trying to decide which therapies are most suitable for you, be guided in the first instance by my comments. All of the therapies listed here have been tried by me or by other M.E. sufferers, and have been proved effective against the symptoms that I have listed under each. However, do not be frightened to try different therapies, or different combinations of them, from those listed here. Follow your own instincts and intuitions faithfully, and try what seems right to you.

Finding an effective treatment depends largely on how vigorously you pursue your aim. Do not forget that no one, as yet, has discovered a treatment that is effective for most patients for most of the time. Therefore it is up to you to seek out those things which will provide a measure of relief from your particular combination of symptoms. Some of the therapies mentioned in this book may work only partially for you, giving only a temporary respite. If this happens, do not be dismayed. Accept the fact that temporary relief is far better than none at all, and use this period of relief to explore other treatments. The next one you try might be the one that does the trick.

When you have found something that is helpful, stick with it. There is no point in abandoning a successful treatment to try another that might be better, but alternatively might fail. Instead add another therapy, which will work hand-in-hand with your successful one, to your routine of treatment. In this way you will gradually build up a network of interlocking treatments which together will alleviate all of your symptoms. Eventually you will reach a point where you are in remission, and only need to use the therapies often enough to maintain your state of health. At this point it would be wise to use them occasionally as a purely preventive measure, to keep you on the straight and narrow path of health.

For a beginner, the world of alternative medicine can seem a strange and complex place. The majority of us were brought up to consider Western medicine the norm. With a little knowledge and effort we can understand why a doctor should prescribe this particular drug for this particular illness, because the whole system is based on sound logical principles. Alternative therapies are often based on ways of thought that are so different from this that they can seem quite ridiculous. However, each of these different systems of thought is perfectly logical and perfectly sensible within its own context. It is only when you compare them with each other that they begin to seem strange.

The system of thought underlying Western medicine is that most ill-health is caused by external influences, such as germs, lack of proper nutrition and so forth. Because we have been taught this since childhood we tend to accept it without questioning it. The philosophy underlying many of the therapies in this book is that most ill-health is caused by internal influences – mental, emotional or spiritual problems which push the body out of its natural healthy balance. At first glance this new idea seems very strange. How can an internal problem cause you to catch flu, or, for that matter, M.E.? It seems much more logical to assume that environmental influences are responsible for disease. But this theory of external cause has one major stumbling block. With every breath of air and every bite of food we are putting germs into our bodies. That is simply a fact of life. Why do some of these germs affect us, and some of them not? How can you go through weeks of winter surrounded by germs of all types without catching anything? And having escaped illness for weeks, why do you suddenly go down with a cold? Something within you must have changed, preventing your body from destroying the germs efficiently. It is reasonable to believe that this internal change emanates from the mental, emotional or even spiritual levels of your being.

There are, no doubt, grains of truth underlying all of the therapies mentioned in this book. They each have something unique to offer. If they also each seem to have something ridiculous within them, we should be very wary of throwing stones. Western medicine is a glass-house containing one supremely ridiculous fact: we only go to doctors when we are ill. To the Chinese, and many other races with systems of medicine far more ancient than our own, this is hysterically absurd. To them, a doctor is responsible for keeping his patients healthy, not for curing them when they are ill, so he sees them when they are well and makes every effort to keep them that way. If one of his patients should fall ill, the doctor's reputation suffers badly and he receives no payment for the duration of the illness. What could be more sensible, more logical or more practical than this? Prevention is absolutely the best way of treating any disease known to man.

As you start to explore alternative therapies you will find yourself encountering many different philosophies. If you are inclined to study them a little, you will soon have your concepts of health and illness turned upside down. As your horizons expand, these new ideas can give a whole new meaning to life. Of course, it is not necessary to know anything at all about the theory behind a therapy to make it work for you. If you are disinclined to study the ideas contained in each system of thought, the therapies will still be enormously helpful.

When trying the therapies, start with those that have the best chance of relieving your worst symptoms. If you do not achieve an alleviation of the problem within a month or so, try another type of treatment. As soon as you have some success, start to work on your lesser problems in the same way. As and when your minor symptoms change, try new treatments, always starting with those that have proved successful in the past. If healing, for example, helped you to overcome your tiredness, then in all probability it will help you with the nausea and coldness as well. Persist in your explorations and you will eventually overcome your illness.

The therapies

Acupuncture and acupressure

Acupuncture and acupressure were two of the first therapies stemming directly from oriental medicine to establish themselves in the West. They are now popular enough to be available in all of the major cities and in many provincial towns too.

The most important writings on acupuncture are a collection of thirty-four books known as the *Nei Ching*. This collection took over 1500 years to complete, with the final chapter being written about 3000 years ago. The acupuncture techniques described in these books were carried out with 'stone piercers' or 'stone borers', but by Neolithic times the Chinese were using needles of bone or bamboo. The discovery of metal marked a major development in the science of acupuncture, and iron, silver and many alloys have all been used to make needles in the past. Today, the acupuncturist uses needles of processed stainless steel.

Originally it was thought that it was the substance the needles were made from which cured disease, but later it was established that it was the method of application which produced such a beneficial effect. It became known that certain points on the skin affected, and perhaps controlled, the working of certain organs of the body. Using needles on these points affected the associated organs, which could be healed of disease by this method.

Underlying acupuncture and acupressure is the theory that two flows of energy, called *yin* and *yang*, exist in the body. These are contained within an overall conception of energy known as the life force or *Ch'i*. These energies are part of everything we do, think or feel. When they are flowing freely, and in balance with each other, these energies produce what we know as health. When a flow is blocked or unbalanced, disease is the result. The Chinese discovered that this vital energy circulates through the body in the same way as blood. The channels it flows in are called meridians.

There are twenty-six major meridians, each associated with an organ or body function, and acupuncture/acupressure points occur where the meridians emerge at the surface of the body. Traditionally there are in excess of 800 of these points, and new ones are being discovered continually. By piercing the skin (acupuncture) or massaging it (acupressure) at these points, the energy flow can be stimulated or sedated. This restores the energy balance within the body, bringing about a functioning equilibrium within the whole being.

Every single point produces a different effect on the energy, and thus in the body, and learning about each of the points and its effect is a lifetime's study. For this reason, the practice of acupuncture is a very complex business and best left to the professionals. Acupressure is much safer to use on yourself, and there are many books on the market which will introduce you to the major pressure points and tell you how to stimulate them correctly.

The main benefits which can come from acupuncture/ acupressure treatment to an M.E. sufferer are pain relief and increased vitality and strength. Individuals for whom it works well also report various minor benefits including improvements in vision and comprehension. I can offer no personal tips for information as I have always been unresponsive to these therapies. Although I have occasionally found acupressure useful for stress relief, I have never experienced any major benefits from either treatment, which puts me in a small minority.

However, I do have enough experience to answer the most common questions about acupuncture. 'Do the needles hurt?' is a frequent one, and the answer is 'No'. Very often you will be entirely unaware that the needle has been inserted until you look. The next question is often, 'What do you feel?' The answer depends entirely on how sensitive you are to the subtle energies of your own body. If you are sensitive in this respect, you may feel a range of responses – warmth, coolness, tingling or a general sensation of what might be called release. The sensations are usually quite pleasant.

In these AIDS-aware days, many people are scared of acupuncture because of the possibility of catching the HIV virus. This fear is entirely groundless. No reputable practitioner would ever use unsterilized needles, and very often the needles will be sterilized in your presence. Feel free to check this with your practitioner. They will fully understand your worries and do everything possible to reassure you.

As far as acupressure is concerned, I can vouch for its effectiveness even though it does not help me personally. I learnt the basics of the technique to use with massage, and over the years many of my friends have benefited from my use of it. It is very simple and usually immediately effective, though it can be briefly painful. This is because instead of a fine needle you are using your finger or thumb to put pressure on a point. Therefore the whole of the surrounding area is pressed and massaged too. If a deep massage is required to stimulate the pressure point fully, this can be uncomfortable for a brief period.

Most people find that if these therapies are going to be helpful, the benefits are obvious very quickly, sometimes immediately after the first session, so finding out whether this therapy is right for you is fairly quick and simple. If, after three or four sessions, you are still feeling no better, then it may be wise to try out some other form of treatment. Acupuncture and acupressure, like all the other therapies, are completely safe in various combinations, but they are particularly harmonious with reflexology and healing.

Autogenic training

Developed by J.H. Schultz in the early part of this century, autogenic training is an unique combination of hypnotic and relaxation techniques. It is often used by sufferers of long-term or chronic sickness, because in the later stages of the therapy the individual can devise exercises which affect those specific areas of the mind and body which are giving trouble. In effect, the therapy is tailored to the precise needs of each individual.

The therapy started almost by accident when some students of Schultz, who were studying autohypnosis (see below), started entering a strange mental state during their practice periods. The state was one of deep physical and mental relaxation and mental clarity. The students reported that after a few minutes of this they emerged refreshed and invigorated, with all fatigue and tension gone. This prompted Schultz to start experimenting further to find out more about the recuperative powers of this state of mind.

The experiments were very successful. The most important discovery, which led directly to the development of autogenic training, was that if the subject concentrated on a positive thought while in this state, improvements in mental and physical well-being came about according to the directions contained in the positive thought. In this way people could gain control of their own energies in a way which had not been known before.

By the 1920s, Schultz had evolved and simplified the technique to create a range of standard exercises to bring harmony to all aspects of mind and body. These are called the Autogenic Standard Series, and form the central core of the therapy. Each exercise involves concentrating passively on a series of mental commands while lying with eyes closed in a quiet room. The exercises have to be practised several times daily, until you can voluntarily shift from a state of high mental or physical arousal to a lower one.

The major drawback to this therapy is the time it takes to master the basic exercises. A person who is healthy in mind and body can take several months to learn the processes fully, and a person who is physically or mentally depleted may find that the learning period has to be extended considerably. Unfortunately, it is only when the basics have been mastered that the individual can start to develop the mental commands which are tailored to their own situation or illness.

Even with this drawback, I would still recommend autogenic training to you. Once learnt it is a simple, safe and effective way to make sure that your mental and physical energies remain relatively free and healthy. What's more, it also makes you realize that you and you alone are responsible for your state of body and mind, which is a fact that we all tend to overlook.

Obviously the positive mental commands concentrated on during the exercises do help, but in the case of M.E. the deep relaxation alone is enough to bring about benefits. Almost everyone who tries a therapy which includes some tuition in relaxation is surprised by the benefits it brings. I suspect that most people think, 'When you are constantly tired and weak, who needs to be relaxed?' The truth is that relaxation refreshes you in mind and body in a way that nothing else can match.

People who have learnt autogenics, autohypnosis or any other form of deep relaxation soon realize that a few minutes of proper relaxing is more refreshing than hours of sleep. In this sense, at least, autogenics can be a highly helpful therapy.

The major benefits of this therapy are the refreshing of physical energy and the renewal of mental concentration and comprehension. Everyone will notice improvements in these areas as they study the technique. Other major symptoms, such as muscular pain, etc., can be controlled, but the degree of control varies from person to person. Once the technique is mastered it can be used to reduce or eliminate many minor symptoms. Altogether it is a very effective therapy if you have the time, energy and will to study it fully.

Autogenics instructors often advertise in the classified section of metropolitan newspapers and magazines. Instructors are unlikely to be widely available in rural areas, but it is possible to teach yourself the basics of the technique from books. Autogenic exercises are completely compatible with every other therapy available.

Aromatherapy

This therapy is one of the most elegant and pleasurable I have ever studied. It is also one of the most consistently successful.

Aromatherapy, as the name suggests, relies on the aroma of natural substances to produce its therapeutic success. The origin of the fragrances can be herbs, woods, spices, flowers or resins, but in every case only the pure oil which gives the substance its natural fragrance is used. This oil, once distilled out, is the essence of the plant or resin it came from, so it is often sold as essential oil as well as aromatherapy oil.

Every practitioner and student of this ancient craft seems to have their own suggestions as to why fragrances should have a medicinal effect. Some reason that the use of these plant essences is akin to herbalism. Some claim that the natural fragrances affect the unconscious mind and thus heal the body. I have met more than one person who believes that the spirit of the plant is captured in its essence, and it is this which heals the user. Whatever the reason for its success, it works well for almost everyone who tries it.

The simplicity of this therapy is its greatest virtue. It can be used at any time and under any circumstances whatsoever. The simplest method of use is to dab a little of the appropriate oil on the inside of your nostrils, so that you are continually inhaling the fragrance. Alternatively, you can place a drop on a radiator, candle or light bulb (before switching it on), which will fill the room with a therapeutic aroma. Adding essential oil to a basic massage oil brings a new dimension to both therapies, and scenting your bath water with a few drops of pure essence produces immediate benefits to mind and body.

Selecting the appropriate oil to counteract your symptoms can be confusing for the beginner. There are dozens of oils and each has a different therapeutic value. From the original dozens, literally thousands of new scents can be developed by combining the oils to enhance their effect. Do not worry about trying to mix complicated combinations at first. Stick to using single oils until you have found ones that work for you, then start combining them in equal proportions. Test these simple mixtures and adjust the combination or proportions according to your own results. In no time at all you will be confidently mixing up all sorts of fragrant brews for yourself, friends and family.

To help you take your first steps in this productive and entertaining therapy, I have prepared a list of oils which many M.E. sufferers find beneficial. Select your first oils from this list, and then add to your collection oils recommended to help with your particular problems. Any aromatherapy book will be helpful in this respect.

Tiredness, weakness, pain and coldness all produce tension, so the first oil you should think about trying is Oil of Lavender, which is a strong relaxant. As I have already noted, relaxation is extremely important as it allows the mind and body to release tensions and toxins and draw in new energy. The light and flowery fragrance of lavender exerts a soothing influence, melting away both physical and mental fatigue. After a bad day, a few drops of this essence in a warm bath prepares you for a night of good, refreshing sleep. Another benefit of lavender is its versatility. It can be mixed with almost any other oil with pleasing results.

Oil of Lemon (note, not Oil of Lemongrass) is one that people tend to shy away from, imagining that it will have a bitter, acidic scent. In fact it is very pleasant, with a fresh, cool fragrance which produces a very calming effect on the mind. Its primary use is to unwind and refresh the mind, though it is also useful to prevent night sweats and fevers. If you mix lemon and lavender, the two scents combine to produce the aromatic equivalent of knock-out drops. In periods of disturbed or unrefreshing sleep, this combination is invaluable. It helps you to sleep well and emerge renewed.

Like lemon, Oil of Peppermint is useful in the prevention of night sweats and fevers, as it has a pronounced cooling effect. However, peppermint is best used in the morning as it is an invigorating scent, an energizer for mind and body. It is also good for any digestive difficulties as it regulates the whole digestive system gently but firmly.

Oil of Basil is another invigorating aroma, but in a slightly different way. It acts to lift the spirits and clear the mind. In a bath it produces a slightly electric tingling sensation which is pleasantly stimulating, but you should be wary of using more than a couple of drops at a time. In larger amounts it can irritate the skin quite painfully. Be a bit careful when mixing basil with other oils as well. It does not combine at all successfully with some of the lighter, more flowery fragrances. It does usually mix well with essences drawn from other herbs or from woods.

Oil of Rosemary is excellent against lethargy and early morning sluggishness. Its clean, sharp fragrance stimulates the mind and body, and prepares you for a new day. Oil of Clary Sage is another good tonic, suitable for use any time in the day. The nutty, floral scent is warming and soothing, and you will probably find that it leaves you feeling pleasantly high and optimistic. Clary sage (note, not ordinary Oil of Sage) is another versatile oil which can be blended with confidence.

Oil of Orange (or Oil of Sweet Orange) is a good addition to your collection because of its all-over helpfulness. It is generally considered to be refreshing and uplifting, and helps to keep you at a mental and physical peak.

Oil of Geranium is a remarkable cleanser of both body and mind, so I would highly recommend its use on those days when you feel slow and unresponsive, as though your system were clogged up. Another benefit of geranium (also called rose geranium) is its effectiveness in harmonizing troubled emotions, so it is useful to keep handy as an antidote to the whole range of emotional problems which can accompany M.E.

Most of the oils you can buy are completely safe to use, though of course none should be taken internally except under professional supervision. However, one or two oils, such as peppermint and basil from the list above, should be used with care as they can irritate the skin. If you are planning to apply the oils directly to your skin, as in a massage, then it is safest to get into the habit of diluting them before use. All of the oils can be diluted with any vegetable oil without losing their therapeutic effect. You can purchase specially blended base oils to dilute them with, but for the ultimate in luxurious skin care, I would suggest that you dilute the essences with Oil of Sweet Almond (Almond Oil), which is extremely beneficial to the skin and available cheaply at most chemists.

Although the oils are fairly widely available through health shops, department stores and other retail outlets, they are quite expensive, which can be a drawback. Often they are cheaper if you buy by mail order. The classified section of most health magazines includes advertisments from suppliers, so it should not be too difficult to locate one. The reason for the expense is that only tiny quantities of oil exist in each plant, so hundreds of plants must be processed to produce each bottle of pure essence.

Some M.E. sufferers consider that there is another drawback to aromatherapy: the relief it provides is temporary and daily treatment may be necessary. To me, this is a short-sighted attitude. Nothing known as yet permanently alleviates M.E. and, until we find something that does, any therapy which provides relief from the symptoms is worthwhile. The relief provided by aromatherapy, and the other treatments, may be short term, but it allows you to think and feel positive for a while, which is a major factor in your favour on a day-to-day basis.

Bach flower remedies

In the year before the First World War, Dr Edward Bach gained his Diploma of Public Health at Cambridge. This was only one of the many qualifications and distinctions gained by him during his long and productive career in medicine. His career embraced both medical practice and research, and he has been credited with excellent work in both fields. However, it was not until his retirement that he began the work which has kept his name in the public eye ever since.

On retiring, Dr Bach turned away from the drugs and surgery that had been his tools as an orthodox physician, and began to experiment with the healing powers of plants and trees. He fully accepted the belief that nature provides everything man needs, and set about finding natural remedies for disease.

His research led him to conclusions that were far in advance of the science of his time. He stated that illness was the result of, or the 'crystallization' of, negative mental attitudes. Now, with our greater understanding of mind and body and how they work together as an inseparable unit, we can start to understand and agree with his belief. Then, it was a revolutionary statement for a supposedly orthodox physician to make.

Having accepted that disease was a psychological rather than a physical problem, Dr Bach realized that treating the physical symptoms of any disease was incorrect. To achieve a complete cure, the psychological weakness had to be rectified. At this point it was natural for him to turn to the plants and trees that he loved in his search for cures of the mind.

Eventually Dr Bach evolved a whole new theory of treatment. He insisted that treating disease was incorrect and taught that the patient's inner self should be treated, as the cause of the illness lay there. In the same way, he insisted that all symptoms should be ignored by the therapist. Instead, the patient's temperament should be examined to uncover the negative mental attitude which had caused the disease. It was this inner dis-ease that had to be treated every time.

Dr Bach listed the major causes of negativity – fear, uncertainty, lack of optimism, etc. – and treated them with preparations made from plants and trees. His method of making these preparations was simple. He picked the appropriate flower and allowed it to stand in water for an hour, in direct sunlight. He found that this process transferred some substance or energy from the flower into the water, which became sparkling and lively. The patient was advised to drink a few drops of this lively water several times a day.

The fact that this therapy has persisted in use, and is becoming increasingly popular, is a testament to its effectiveness. The original thirty-eight flower remedies isolated by Dr Bach are still in use, and they are still prepared according to his original method.

The benefits of this therapy are its simplicity and effectiveness. However, it does not work for everyone. If it is successful for you, you will find that the remedies alleviate or cure all of the mental and emotional symptoms of M.E., and can radically improve your physical state. This physical improvement seems to come about because the therapy drastically reduces stress levels, which gives the body a chance to heal itself. The drawbacks are that the therapy is not widely available compared with, for instance, acupuncture. Also, unless you are very experienced at diagnosing your own emotional states, it is wiser to go to a professional practitioner for diagnosis and treatment. You can study the subject from books if no practitioner is available to you, and advertisements in health magazines are a good place to locate suppliers.

Colonic irrigation

This is a rather odd therapy that has had bursts of popularity over the years, but has never become established on a wide scale. Perhaps this is because it has a very limited usage in orthodox medicine, and its claims as an alternative therapy have never, as far as I am aware, been substantiated. It has been suggested as a suitable treatment for M.E., so it deserves to be included here.

Colonic irrigation is a standard part of the regime in some health spas and naturopathic clinics. Based on the same principles of hygiene and comfort as the enema, colonic irrigation requires more complicated equipment and affects a larger area of the body. The procedure is simple. For a varying period (usually thirty to forty-five minutes) water at body temperature is injected into the rectum. The water flows out again via a two-way tube. Irrigation is more effective than an enema because it reaches above the normal defecation area, into the descending and transverse colon. As the water is washed in and out it detaches any old faecal matter adhering to these areas.

Usually colonic irrigation will only be recommended after

two or three days of fasting, so that all faeces and digestive residues have passed out of the colon. This is not the only limitation to its use. Conditions such as diverticulitis, certain types of colitis and malignant growths can be vastly aggravated by this therapy. Normally it should also be avoided in cases of greatly reduced vitality. As M.E. reduces vitality to a large degree, it is questionable whether this therapy would be advisable for the majority of sufferers.

There is one side-effect of colonic irrigation which is usually considered a problem but may be of benefit to M.E. patients. During irrigation many of the normal digestive bacteria are washed out of the colon. As I have already noted, *Candida* bacteria reside in the digestive system and can cause problems for some sufferers when they get out of control. Washing out these masses of bacteria may be a good treatment for people who have severe problems in this area. Also, irrigation is effective in controlling constipation, which can be of great benefit, but there are simpler ways of achieving the same result.

Usually this treatment is prescribed for chronic conditions in which proper elimination of body wastes may be vitally important – catarrh, gastric troubles, skin disorders, etc. It should always be accompanied by strict dietary control.

There seems little logical reason to put colonic irrigation high on your list of appropriate therapies. Having said that, I must add that a few people have found it helpful, and throughout its long history the therapy has always had its devotees. Mae West, for example, swore by it as a necessity for health and beauty, and often practised it daily.

If you decide to try colonic irrigation, do so only under the direct supervision of qualified medical personnel.

Diet

There is no suggestion whatsoever that diet causes or can cure M.E. However, during the illness your body may require different foods in different amounts from your normal intake. Adjusting your diet can help to prevent or remedy a worsening of your symptoms. If your body does require different foods from normal you may experience cravings and aversions or just a general dissatisfaction with what you are eating. These feelings are your body's way of telling you of what it needs to function properly, so it is usually wise to give in to them.

Aversions are the simplest to spot, and should always be obeyed without question. To take a common example, alcohol is a substance to which many sufferers develop an aversion. This aversion is easy to abide by because drinking even small amounts of alcohol can produce an immediate worsening of all symptoms. Why this should happen is not known, but happen it does. Obviously your metabolism is no longer in a fit state to deal with alcohol, so it is wise to cut it out altogether. You will find that your tolerance for alcohol gradually increases as you get better.

Tea is another common aversion. Like many people I was a regular tea drinker until I discovered that my several cups a day were worsening the illness. As decaffeinated coffee produces no ill effects, I assume it is the stimulants in tea which are harmful to a weakened and overstressed system. As an experiment I tried decaffeinated tea for a while, and found that it produced no ill effects. Unfortunately it made such a revolting brew that it was worse than drinking no tea at all.

There will be some aversions which are peculiar to yourself – foods and drinks which badly affect you and you alone. These are easy to discover. Within minutes, or at most an hour, of eating them you will start to feel bad. If you think that something is affecting you in this way, you can make sure by carrying out the following simple test: eat normally but avoid the suspect food for a day or two. Next morning, eat nothing for three to four hours after getting up. Then eat a normal-sized portion of the suspect food. If it is bad for you, you will feel worse almost immediately, and you should avoid that food from then on.

Using this simple exclusion test I discovered that salt and vinegar crisps and pickled onions were extremely detrimental to my well-being. Either of these things would send my temperature rocketing up and make me feel dizzy and nauseous. It may be that prior to my illness I had an allergy to these things, but it was so mild that it never gave me any real problem. With my system weakened by illness, any allergy would become much more obvious and would be a serious strain on my defences, complicating all the other symptoms.

Cravings are sometimes harder to deal with because giving

in to them indiscriminately can cause problems in the long term. A frequent craving is for sugary foods. Sometimes your body's demands for sweet things can last for weeks at a time. If you give in to it over a lengthy period, you may be causing weight problems for yourself in the future. Try things like sugar-free chewing gum, which tastes sweet but is very low in calories. This can help you satisfy the craving without setting up problems later on. Alternatively, sweet fruits and vegetables like bananas and carrots can help to satisfy you. If only the real sweetness of sugar will satisfy you, remember that pure honey is a healthier substitute for white sugar in drinks and puddings.

As with aversions, you will probably have cravings that are entirely personal to you. My main failing in this regard was an unquenchable hunger for cold rice pudding. For a period of some weeks when I was ill it became an important feature of my diet because I could not stand the thought of other foods. I was a little unsure whether this was a good thing at first, because of all the sugar and fats it contains. Then I reasoned that it had to be better than no food at all, and ate it to my heart's content. Just to satisfy my conscience about healthy eating, I made it with brown rice to keep up my fibre intake. As a general rule, satisfy your cravings where possible, but bear in mind your overall diet and do not allow excesses of sugar, fats or stimulants to continue for long.

Your overall diet plan should provide enough of every type of food to fulfil your body's needs. Do not forget that even though you are doing very little, your body is constantly working hard to throw off your illness, so it is important that it gets enough food.

Many people find that a macrobiotic or wholefood diet is very helpful. These diets, high in natural nutrients, provide everything your body needs and eliminate most artificial additives. Also, the high fibre content in brown bread, brown rice, wholewheat pasta and so on, helps to maintain regularity in your digestive system and bowel, which can prevent constipation and other unwanted complications.

When to eat is another important question. Too many people eat little or nothing in the early part of the day, and make up for it later on with a big meal. This may suit you perfectly when you are healthy, but a fast-and-feast pattern is devastating when you are unwell. It places a strain on your entire system, one which you could well do without and can easily avoid. Try to get into the habit of eating at least three small meals a day, at equally spaced intervals. By doing this you are regularly giving your body the fuel it needs to fight off the illness and function efficiently. You will soon notice the benefits of this alteration if you keep to a regular routine of eating. You will feel stronger, warmer and more alert, and will be more resistant to a relapse.

Excercise

The simple answer to the question of exercise is: don't. In the past doctors have often misguidedly ordered patients to exercise to relieve muscular pain and stiffness. It usually makes the condition chronic. Even people who suffer little from the muscular problems associated with M.E. will find that exercise is a sure and certain way to achieve a relapse.

When you are in a bout of illness, avoid all exercise whenever possible. During convalescence, exercise becomes both necessary and beneficial.

As soon as you feel well enough to think about getting out and about, start to take a little exercise regularly. A daily stroll to the park or shops is great, but do not expect to be able to do this immediately. Start with trips into and around your own garden, or somewhere equally close at hand. As your strength returns, gradually make more ambitious journeys. Always remain aware of your resources and never tire yourself to the danger point of inviting a relapse.

The benefits of exercise are many. Mentally it gives you a lift, making you feel part of the world once more. Fresh air and a change of scenery can do more to keep you alert and optimistic than any amount of therapy. Physically the exercise helps to cleanse and tone your body, helping it to get rid of wastes effectively and maintain a healthy balance. You will find that your sleep and appetite improve, and you will generally feel less feeble.

Avoid all violent or strenuous activities until you are sure, beyond a shadow of a doubt, that you can cope with them. Be prepared to stop whatever you are doing as soon as you start to feel that sinking, draining sensation which tells you that your

strength is ebbing. Above all, remember the golden rule: if in
doubt, don't.

Healing

The various names of spiritual healing, psychic healing and faith
healing are all ultimately misleading. If healing needs any further
description at all, the word 'natural' should be placed in front
of it. Healing is the natural ability of one person to restore health
in another.

Healing has existed for as long as mankind and is entirely
independent of faith, psychic perceptions or spiritual beliefs.
It is simply an exchange of energy from the healer to the patient
which increases the patient's vitality. This leads to a quicker,
sometimes instantaneous, recovery from illness or injury.

Most of us have experienced this type of energy exchange
in everyday life. I am sure that you have come across people
whose presence left you feeling uplifted, happy and full of energy.
Conversely, you have probably also met people who leave you
feeling drained and dispirited. In each case there has been an
exchange of vital energy. The vital energy in each of us is not
a static thing. It changes according to mood and environment,
and flows from person to person. Sadness, tiredness, depression
and a host of other negative feelings all allow our vital energy
to drain away, and prevent it from being replenished from the
normal internal sources. When this happens, the person will
unconsciously draw vitality from external sources to try to regain
their own balance. These external sources are often other people.

Healers are people who either have a strong natural link with
their own inner source of energy, or have worked and practised
to develop such a link. Once this link is functioning properly,
the healer has an almost inexhaustible supply of vital energy
which can be shared with anyone in need. This vitality can be
directed to the patient to help them overcome whatever internal
or external factors have put them out of touch with their own
source of strength. This then frees the natural healing powers
of the patient's mind and body to correct any imbalances.

Healing is a very simple therapy. You only have to give the
briefest explanation of your problems to the healer, often none
at all, then he or she will start the treatment. Usually the healer

likes to make contact with you by putting their hands on your shoulders, head or the problem area. Some healers prefer to hold their hands a few inches away from your body. As they start to send energy to you, you will probably feel a sensation of intense warmth spreading from their hands to your body. Occasionally, depending on the healer, the sensation might be of coolness or tingling. The treatment usually lasts for a minimum of five minutes, and can go on for up to fifteen minutes or longer if the practitioner feels you are badly in need of energy. During the treatment you will start to feel relaxed, happy and calm, and these feelings can stay with you for days after your session.

At various times I have been both healer and patient, though usually the former, and so I have a fairly comprehensive understanding of this therapy. I recommend it without hesitation to sufferers of all illness, regardless of the nature of their complaint. I have never seen or heard of a case in which the patient did not benefit from the treatment in some way. The only limitation to the power of this vital energy is the skill, insight and experience of the healer. If you do not respond at first, find another practitioner.

Many times I have had people coming to see me who looked awful – tense, drawn, tired and ill – but as they walked out after the treatment, their whole appearance had changed. In some cases they actually gave every indication of being healthy once more, and in every case their faces showed a glow of returning vitality. This outward change is only the echo of a more important inner healing. Within a period of hours, and sometimes minutes, even chronic conditions such as kidney failure, tumours and wasting diseases can be relieved by a proper application of the vital force of healing. Occasionally they are cured outright. I know from experience that these 'miracle' healings definitely do happen, but they are comparatively rare. Like most other therapies, healing has a cumulative effect over a period of time and a number of treatments. Expect to have to visit your healer a few times before big improvements start to become obvious. Even so, you will find little improvements coming about from the start, so the regular visit to your healer will probably become an enjoyable outing.

Healing is very widely available, and very often the healer

will be willing to come to you if you are not able to travel to them. You may, however, have to pay their travelling expenses. Most faith and spiritual healers believe that their talent is a gift to be shared freely with the rest of mankind, so they do not charge for their services. Increasingly, though, healers are coming to realize that their talent is no gift. It is purchased at the cost of long study and training, just the same as the skills of a therapist in any other field. And like all other therapists, the practitioner has the right to charge patients for this skill and experience. Some healers charge around £30 per treatment, which I feel is a little excessive, whilst others keep their charges in line with comparable therapies such as homoeopathy. Expect to pay around £10 to £15 per treatment from a good healer if you cannot find one locally who gives their services free.

If you have the money to pay for healing, then it is probably wise to do so. This therapy is only as good as the individual practitioner, and a professional is more likely to be effective than a well-meaning amateur. It is not uncommon to find healers who give their services freely and are dedicated to high ideals, but who lack any real talent or training for healing. Persevere in your search for a reputable practitioner. When you find an effective healer the benefits to your health will be immediate and striking.

Herbalism

Herbal medicine is best described as the art and science of restoring health by using remedies originating from plants. These remedies, referred to as herbs though they can come from any type of plant, have been shown in many cases to be just as powerful as orthodox drugs but free from the possible toxic side-effects of drug therapy. Many qualified physicians are now studying herbalism to use alongside or instead of orthodox drugs.

There are records of this type of medicine being in use since at least 1500 years before the time of Christ, so it is certainly one of the best established of alternative therapies. However, it is also perhaps the most complex, and treatment for serious complaints should be left exclusively to the professional practitioner.

When selecting an appropriate treatment for you, herbalists

will tend to look first at your symptoms, but will also examine your temperament and mental state. The medicine they prescribe will take all of these factors into account. This means that treatment will vary widely from person to person, so it is of little use to suggest here herbs which might be beneficial to you.

Qualified herbalists can be difficult to find, and pursuing a course of treatment can be expensive. If you have had success with other plant-based therapies (aromatherapy, Bach flower remedies, etc.) it could be worth your while to invest in a trial of this type of treatment. Ask in your local health shop if they can refer you to a good local herbalist, or check the advertisements in health magazines to locate a practitioner. Herbalism should be quite safe for use in combination with the other therapies, but if you are also receiving homoeopathic treatment or taking any other course of treatment which involves ingesting therapeutic substances, let all your therapists know exactly what you are doing.

Homoeopathy

Homoeopathy is sometimes hard for people to accept as a valid system of medicine, for two reasons. The first is that its basic theory is completely opposed to medicine as we know and understand it. For example, an orthodox (or allopathic) doctor will usually prescribe drugs that counteract the symptoms the patient is experiencing: if you have a fever, the doctor will give you something to cool you down. This seems perfectly logical and straightforward. A homoeopathic doctor would approach the problem from the opposite direction. Instead of prescribing a cooling medicine, he would give you a tiny dose of a substance which in large quantities would cause the type of fever you are experiencing. This makes homoeopathy difficult to understand for people brought up on allopathic principles of treatment.

The second reason for the lack of acceptance of homoeopathy is the medicines themselves: the more they are diluted, the stronger they become. In many common preparations the original substance has been diluted to the point where the final tablet contains only one part per million of the substance. As we are all trained to think that power is measurable by its quantity or volume, this process of dilution seems to be counterproductive.

However, before dismissing this therapy out of hand, there are two facts which should be noted. They are that this therapy has been in existence since the eighteenth century and that it is one of the most widely available and consistently popular of all alternative therapies. These facts testify to its effectiveness over a long period of years. We may not know how or why it works, but hundreds of thousands of people have found that it does.

Homoeopathic remedies are drawn from the animal, vegetable and mineral kingdoms. The effect of each on the human system is thoroughly investigated before it is approved for use. There are hundreds, or perhaps thousands, of approved remedies and more are being discovered all the time. This means that homoeopathic practitioners have a vast selection of potential remedies to choose from. To make their selection they will require detailed descriptions of all your symptoms, and they will also take into account your temperament and, if applicable, your occupation, lifestyle and daily habits. This can make examinations hard work for the patient but they are usually worthwhile. Most people who have persisted with homoeopathic treatment report major or minor benefits, but they vary from person to person. There does not seem to be one particular area which is reliably helped by this therapy.

Although all homoeopathic treatments are completely safe, it is such a complex system that selecting your own remedies is really out of the question. All practitioners have to have qualified as orthodox doctors first in order to qualify as homoeopaths; therefore they can be difficult to find. Most sizeable towns will have at least one homoeopathic doctor, so keep asking around until you find one in your area. Be prepared to have a lengthy wait before you see the doctor. They are so much in demand that there is usually a long list of patients to be seen before your appointment comes round.

Hydrotherapy

The term 'hydrotherapy' covers a vast range of techniques, all of which feature water as the main therapeutic agent. Many of these techniques are complicated and/or expensive, but there are two which are suitable for home use and can help all M.E.

sufferers. The first and most important is the hot bath.

Technically the temperature for a hot bath can be anywhere from 38°C (100°F) upwards. In practice, you will want to have the water a lot warmer than that. The main benefit of a hot bath is the sweating which it induces, and 38°C is too cool to do you much good in this regard. However, having the water too hot is counter-productive. Remember that you are going to be in the bath for at least ten minutes and perhaps for as long as an hour, so select a temperature which will be comfortable over this period of time.

Having prepared your bath, the only other thing you have to do is get in and enjoy it. Wallow in the water, moving it around all parts of your body. Immerse yourself totally if possible – if not, then dip all parts regularly. Once you have started to sweat, then relax until you feel that you have had enough. When you get out, dry yourself well and wrap up to prevent yourself chilling too fast. Try to cool off gradually, and always rest for at least an hour after emerging. It is best to bathe in the evening so that you can fall into bed when you have cooled off a little. A glass of water before bed is an excellent idea, to make sure you replace the fluid lost through sweating.

The first benefit of a hot bath is the obvious one. You get hot. This must not be underestimated. If you have been suffering from coldness, the relief of warmth is a blessing in itself. Apart from this, the bath will improve your circulation, bring you to a state of deep relaxation, and enable your body to sweat out many toxins and wastes produced by the disease. Sweating in a bath seems to help prevent the recurrence of night sweats and fevers. Generally you will find that a hot bath makes you feel better all over, reducing most of your symptoms to a noticeable degree.

Combining the hot bath with other therapies is an excellent idea. Herbs and minerals added to the bath have an immediate effect as they are easily absorbed through the open pores of the skin. Personally, I think that aromatherapy is the best, and simplest, addition to hydrotherapy. The two combine luxuriously, enhancing one another enormously. It really does give a whole new meaning to the idea of bathing.

Russian, Turkish, and sauna baths have exactly the same therapeutic effect as hot baths. If you have not tried these more exotic types of baths before, it is wise to stay in them for short periods only during your first few visits. You can gradually extend the length of your stay in subsequent visits, when you have adjusted to the intense heat.

The second hydrotherapy technique of use to M.E. sufferers is the neutral bath. As the name suggests, this is a bath of neutral, or blood, temperature. The main benefit of this type of bath is the deep relaxation it produces. This eliminates mental and physical tension and fatigue. Neutral baths can and should last longer than hot baths, so you must remember to keep adjusting the temperature in case you get too cold. Again, adding herbs, minerals or aromatherapy oils increases the therapeutic value.

There is one other hydrotherapy technique which may be of use to a minority of sufferers. If you have severe muscular pain and the swelling which sometimes accompanies this condition, then alternating baths will probably help you. The technique is perfectly safe and simple, but it can be quite a shock to the system as it relies on alternating hot and cold water in a rapid sequence.

If it is your leg(s) which require treatment, then sit on the edge of the bath with your legs in the bath. If it is any part of your upper body that is to be treated, then it will probably be simpler to undress completely and sit in the bath.

Once you are comfortable, start the treatment by running hot water over the affected muscles. Using a shower head for this is the best way, but bowls of water poured quickly will do almost as well. The water should be as hot as you can comfortably bear. After two, or at most three, minutes of hot water, switch immediately to very cold water, and run this over the affected part for thirty seconds. Then switch back to hot again for another two to three minutes, followed by cold again, for thirty seconds. Repeat the hot/cold sequence once more to complete the treatment.

You will find that this treatment will reduce all swelling and inflammation very rapidly. Some sufferers report that it also reduces pain considerably for reasonable periods of time.

All of these hydrotherapy techniques are completely safe for regular home use. They will combine well with any other therapies you may be trying.

Hypnosis and autohypnosis

Many people still hold the outdated idea that hypnotists are Svengali-type characters, whose only aim in life is to reduce the entire population to helpless zombies. Nothing could be further from the truth. The vast majority of hypnotists are responsible professionals who have mastered an excellent technique for helping people to help themselves.

Hypnosis can be defined as an altered state of consciousness in which the subject's logical, critical mind is bypassed. This state can only be achieved with the subject's consent. At all times they remain aware of and in control of their responses.

Being in an hypnotic trance is rather like being on the borderland between sleep and waking. You feel warm and comfortable and drowsy. While in this state your logical mind fades into the background, so you are very uncritical of anything you hear. If the hypnotist says, 'You are feeling well. You are feeling strong. You feel no pain', then your mind accepts this as the truth. Because your criticial faculty is 'sleeping', you truly believe the ideas suggested to you by the hypnotist. Once your mind has fully accepted the suggestion that you are well and fit, you immediately start to feel better. This mind over matter effect is very real. Through the use of hypnosis your own unconscious becomes a strong ally in your struggle for health. By having the right suggestions accepted by the unconscious you can reduce or eliminate all of your symptoms.

Regular visits to a hypnotist can prove time consuming and expensive, but if you already know from experience that hypnosis works for you then it is a worthwhile investment. Alternatively, you can learn to hypnotize yourself quite quickly and cheaply, and produce excellent results in the privacy of your own home.

Autohypnosis, as self-hypnosis is called, can easily be learnt from books and tapes. Once you have mastered the basic techniques you can prepare hypnotic suggestions which will get your unconscious mind working to eliminate your particular problems. It will probably take a little time and effort to get it right, but even when you are just starting to practise, you will be benefiting from the therapy. One of the by-products of the hypnotic state is mental and physical relaxation. This relaxation is extraordinarily helpful. You emerge from it feeling as though you have just had a deep and refreshing sleep.

Unfortunately, hypnosis does not work for everyone, and as a therapy it is only as good as the practitioner who uses it. So, try autohypnosis first, preferably from a tape which teaches you about it by putting you into an hypnotic trance. If this is helpful, consider consulting a practitioner. They are widely available and advertise in most magazines and newspapers, but ask among your friends for a personal recommendation – word of mouth is the most reliable advertisement. Hypnotic or autohypnotic therapy is safe in combination with any other therapy, but is enhanced by meditation and by the yoga exercises explained later.

Kinesiology

The techniques of this therapy are most widely known under the name 'Touch for health', which was devised by chiropractic doctors for use by lay people. It is perhaps the simplest method of preventive health care available.

Touch for health is not used for diagnosing or treating specific illnesses. It is used to discover and correct bodily imbalances of any kind. Correcting imbalances ensures that the body functions well and is able to heal itself should the need arise. The simple testing procedure isolates those parts of the body which are not working efficiently, and can show which thoughts, environmental influences or diet substances are responsible for the imbalance. It can also show you which things will best return your body to a state of natural harmony.

Anyone can learn to administer the test procedure. The theory is that each of the twelve major body systems – stomach, lungs, pancreas, etc – is closely related to certain muscles. Any system which is weakened or diseased will show as a weakness in the related muscles. Therefore, testing the muscles for simple physical strength gives a clear indication of internal functions.

What is really remarkable about this technique is the way in which you discover what has caused any imbalance and then isolate a cure for it. A weak muscle will immediately grow weaker if a substance which the body finds harmful is placed in the mouth. Conversely, the muscle will immediately strengthen if a beneficial substance is placed in the mouth. This sounds quite straightforward, but you really have to experience the dramatic effect to comprehend fully how effective this technique can be. Within minutes you can test all the foods in your diet, and find out which are harmful and which are helpful. You can also find out which vitamins, diet supplements, dietary changes or any other form of treatment will help you. You can use this technique to demonstrate clearly your internal reaction to absolutely anything. For M.E. sufferers, knowing which things are acting against the body and weakening it can help to prevent or cure the relapses which occur from time to time, seemingly out of the blue.

Although it is possible to learn this technique from books, it is far better to attend one of the short instructional courses held regularly all over the country. Under the guidance of a trained instructor you will see the technique come to life in an amazing way. The basic course does not qualify you to practise as a therapist, but it does give you an adequate foundation for the use of the technique on friends and family. Unfortunately you cannot test yourself, so you will have to arrange for a friend to help you out with the diagnosis. After you have shown your friends what can be done with this therapy, I am sure that you will have people queueing up to be tested, so arranging for one of them to test you in return should be no problem.

If you want to try this technique without going through the basic course, try to find a qualified practitioner near you. They are usually quite difficult to find as they rarely seem to advertise. Ask around, particularly in your local health shop. They may well have heard of a practitioner in your area.

Massage

A good massage stimulate the muscles just as effectively as a workout, so massage should be treated with the same caution as exercise.

For people whose symptoms include muscular pain, massage is a definite 'Don't'. Although it may help to relieve the pain at first (but certainly not always), it will cause the symptoms to become more intense in the following hours or days. It can even cause degeneration into a chronic state.

If you suffer little from muscular pain and have been

accustomed to receiving regular treatment from a masseur before your illness, then it may be helpful to continue. During the massage you may find that particular areas or muscles are feeling tender. If so, ask your practitioner to avoid these areas altogether.

If you have never had a massage before, then do not try this therapy during a bout of illness. In convalescence, if you are free of all muscular problems, it can be helpful.

The main benefits of massage are relaxation and stress relief, though it also helps with circulation and lymph drainage. It is widely available and can be combined with aromatherapy and hydrotherapy with excellent results.

Meditation

Strictly speaking, this is a discipline rather than a therapy, but as it has distinct therapeutic effects it deserves to be mentioned here.

Basically, meditation is the art of making the mind still. All of the thoughts and feelings, hopes, fears and desires which occupy your mind in most of your waking hours are let go, so that the mind becomes peaceful and calm. This switching off of all the day-to-day agitations of thought produces physical, mental and emotional relaxation. You emerge from the meditative state feeling renewed: calm, strong, refreshed and in control.

The only drawback with meditation is that it can be difficult to learn. Many people find that just as they achieve a degree of stillness, an idea appears from nowhere and their mind chases after it in fast and furious thought. Only patience and perseverance can cure this problem. There are no short-cuts to mastery of the technique. Every time your mind dashes off in a new direction, gently but firmly end the thought and return your mind to the stillness. You may find at first that the stillness, which is empty of all thought, is very difficult to hold on to. If this is the case, select one thought or feeling to concentrate on and keep returning your mind to that during practice periods. Concentrating on one thing only is a stepping-stone to concentrating on nothing. At this stage many people find that concentrating on their breathing is an excellent aid, whilst others prefer to focus their attention on an imaginary flower, a ball of light or any other comfortable image.

Trying to learn to meditate whilst in a bout of illness complicates the whole process. If you want to try this therapy, wait until you are reasonably free of all mental symptoms. This will give you the best chance of learning it quickly and well. However, recognize the fact that it is going to be weeks or months before you feel able to meditate easily, and be prepared to invest the necessary time and energy.

Once you have mastered the basics you will find that meditation is an ongoing process. The more you do it, the more you get from it. Mental and physical problems fade away as the meditation brings you into contact with deeper and deeper levels of your own mind. Eventually you reach the point of feeling that while meditating you are in touch with the very centre of your being. This releases a flow of strength and vitality which has to be felt to be believed.

Once mastered, meditation will stand you in good stead for the rest of your life. In time it will balance and strengthen all of the subtle energies of mind, body and spirit, paving the way for good health. 'In time' is, unfortunately, the operative phrase. As a therapy, meditation is all about long-term goals and benefits, so it is best to consider this as a background therapy and seek other treatments for more immediate relief.

Reflexology

Reflexology, which is simply massage of the hands and feet, has become one of the most popular alternative therapies now that different systems of medicine have caught the imagination of the public at large. Zone therapy, as this treatment is also known, is used as a means of bringing the patient back to a harmonious state of mind and body. Reflexologists believe that health is a direct result of this harmony, which cannot exist if any part of the intricate mechanism that is a human being is maladjusted.

No one can say for sure how or where the reflex method originated. One of the most popular theories is that it came to the West from China, where it existed alongside and was used with acupuncture. The fact that there are several important similarities between these two therapies tends to support the theory of an oriental origin, but reflexology is also known to have been used by the natives of Kenya and by some American Indian tribes. Whatever its origin, reflexology as it is currently used stands as a supreme example of an alternative therapy. It is a simple, safe procedure; it involves the patient in their own healing; it is an excellent diagnostic tool and it is equally effective as a preventive and a curative therapy.

The theory of reflexology is very straightforward. Every part of the body is linked, via the nervous system and the subtle energies, to a particular area of the hands and feet. When this area is stimulated by massage, the corresponding organ is affected. This is considered to be a natural reflex, hence the name. The fundamental therapeutic principle is one of releasing tension, thus bringing about a full blood flow to the dis-eased parts, but the massage also stimulates the subtle energies to revitalize and repair the affected area.

Because this reflex link works both ways, ill-health in any part of the body will show clearly in the corresponding reflex zone on the hand or foot. A skilful reflexologist can often diagnose problems before they are fully formed in the body, which is an invaluable aid in preventive health care. Whenever an organ is not functioning correctly, the associated reflex zone will become tender and sensitive to pressure. The discomfort varies according to the severity of the problem, so the patient's help is often asked for to give feedback about changes in the nature or strength of the discomfort. As soon as the pain in a particular area eases off, the corresponding organ is back in a state of good health.

Reflexology helps M.E. sufferers in a number of ways. It always produces relaxation, which amounts to a therapy in itself, but it also aids most of the bodily systems to function efficiently. Digestion and the elimination of wastes are always normalized by zone therapy, as are lymph drainage, breathing and circulation. Other benefits, of which there can be many, vary according to both patient and practitioner.

Finding a practitioner is simple as they are widely available, but finding a good one can be more problematic. Ask whether the practitioner has been trained in either the Ingham or the Bayly technique, as these are the most effective forms of the therapy. The only other guide-line which is of any use is experience. If your session of reflexology is painful, or leaves you feeling drained or ill, find another practitioner. A good practitioner is often sensitive enough to be able to establish a strong rapport with his or her patients, so feeling comfortable and at ease with the therapist is sometimes an indication that the therapy will eventually be of help to you. Benefits should be noticeable from the first session onwards, but they will accumulate over a period of time with each subsequent session.

Reflexology is very simple, but the reflex zones themselves are quite complex. If you wish to invest some time and energy in learning the basics of the technique, you will be able to treat yourself on a daily basis or whenever you feel the need. Even if you would prefer to treat yourself, I would advise at least one session with a professional practitioner so that you can see and feel how it works in practice. This could make a vital difference to your newly acquired skills, as there is no way in which a book can explain the sensitivity that a good practitioner possesses.

This therapy is perfectly safe and compatible with all others. I have found that combining it with aromatherapy or healing produces particularly striking results.

Relaxation

As I have noted again and again the benefits of relaxation, it seems sensible to offer a relaxation technique so that you can try this simple therapy for yourself.

Lie on your back on the floor, and breathe in and out deeply a few times, just to prepare yourself. Then focus your attention on the toes of your right foot. Become aware of your toes as intensely as possible. Then breathe in deeply and clench your toes as tightly as you can, tensing up all the muscles. Hold this for a second, then breathe out slowly, relaxing your toes at the same time. Repeat this for the toes of the left foot. Then return your attention to your right foot. Breathe in deeply and clench the muscles of the whole foot as tightly as possible. Hold this for a second, then breathe out and relax. Repeat this for the left foot. Then progress slowly up the body doing exactly the same thing to every muscle. Work right the way up your body, starting with the calves, then progressing to the thighs, the lower back, the stomach, the upper back, the chest, the arms, the forearms, the hands and fingers and finally the neck, scalp and face. Remember to breathe properly as you tense and relax the muscles.

Doing this exercise properly will produce a sensation of warmth and heaviness in the muscles, and you will feel comfortably relaxed all over. This technique can be combined with any other therapy in perfect safety. Obviously, if you are suffering with severe muscular problems it is not wise to try this method of relaxation. Instead, experiment with hydrotherapy, autohypnosis or yoga breathing as a basis of your relaxation.

Many people do not fully realize the role that tension plays in illness. A tense body cannot heal itself effectively. Tension inhibits most of the body's systems, including circulation, lymph drainage, digestion, elimination of wastes, immune responses, recuperation and regeneration. The vicious circle of illness which produces tension which maintains illness which produces more tension has to be broken if the patient's natural healing mechanisms are to be allowed to overcome the disease. Therefore regular relaxation is a necessity for health of both body and mind and should be included in any routine of therapy.

Royal jelly

Thanks to the ever increasing popularity of this health and beauty treatment, many people now know that royal jelly is a thick off-white liquid produced by bees to feed their queen. What is less well known is the phenomenally wide range of illnesses and complaints which can be alleviated with regular doses of this substance. Royal Jelly is already known to be one of the most nutritious natural foods ever discovered, but reports of scientific investigations into its effects suggest that it is also one of the most potent natural medicines known to man.

In the early days, research into this substance was painfully slow. Royal jelly is only produced in tiny amounts at certain times of year, so collecting enough to experiment with was an arduous task for the scientists. Since the 1960s, scientific and medical interest, coupled with increasing public demand, has encouraged bee-keepers to develop new techniques which trick the bees into producing much larger quantities of royal jelly. This causes the bees no harm whatsoever. Now royal jelly is freely available, there is a constant flow of new and exciting reports about its effect on the human system.

For many years it has been known that royal jelly increases fertility and virility; improves the quality of hair, skin and nails; cleanses the blood; improves circulation and aids the efficient disposal of body wastes. The new reports being issued now show that it has an even more dramatic effect: it is an effective treatment for heart disease; it reduces cholesterol levels and prevents blocked arteries; it prevents and cures stomach ulcers and every other stress-related complaint; it is one of the most efficient natural disinfectants and has anti-fungal and anti-microbial properties; it can relieve even the most severe arthritic and rheumatic conditions; it is a potent diuretic; it improves the absorption of nutrients; it is an effective treatment for depression and neurotic states; it relieves eczema and most other skin complaints; and finally, to bring this list to a very premature end, it has been shown to be effective against cancer in mice, though no human trials have yet been reported.

With an immense weight of scientific evidence in support of royal jelly, it is very surprising that it is still largely ignored by the medical profession. Part of the reason for this lack of acceptance is that we actually know very little about how royal jelly works. In fact, we do not even know entirely what it is made up of. Analysis shows that 96 per cent of the substance is composed of an effective combination of vitamins, minerals and amino acids, all of which are necessary for good health. The other 4 per cent is a complete mystery as it continues to defy every attempt at analysis.

Another reason for its lack of medical usage is that its effect is not consistent. Doctors are trained to expect that a drug will affect the great majority of individuals in a way that is consistent from person to person. Royal jelly does not do this. It affects each individual differently, according to their own needs, harmonizing and balancing their mental and physical systems. If it is given to a patient with high blood-pressure, it brings their blood-pressure down. If it is given to a patient with low blood-pressure, it pushes their blood-pressure up. In every case it normalizes the body, bringing natural functions to a peak of efficiency. Doctors seem very reluctant to accept that this is a treatment which reacts differently according to the needs of the individual patient.

The doubts of the medical profession could be accepted as logical if royal jelly were a potentially dangerous treatment, but it is not. It is a safe, gentle, natural remedy that has never been known to cause any unpleasant side-effects. This being the case, you would imagine that doctors would be delighted to have found such an effective treatment for such a wide range of common ailments. I hope that as the evidence continues to mount, more doctors will put aside their preconceived ideas of what a drug is and how it should work, and accept royal jelly as a valid and valuable addition to their armoury of treatments.

For M.E. sufferers, royal jelly can help in a variety of ways. Among the most important are relief from muscular problems, greater energy and stamina and greater mental alertness. Most of the other symptoms respond equally well. In my own case I experienced a dramatic lessening of muscular pain, and over a period of weeks I regained a degree of mental clarity which I had not had since the illness started. I have seen sufferers who were confined to bed or a wheelchair up and around again in a matter of weeks. One lady, who had been in constant pain for four years, was soon free of major difficulties and told me, 'I keep thinking that I mustn't do things because of the pain, and then I remember that my legs don't hurt any more. It's marvellous!' The vast majority of sufferers who have tried it report physical and mental improvements which have given them a new lease of life.

If you decide to try treating yourself with royal jelly, then be prepared to give it an extended trial. For a normal healthy person, using royal jelly as a preventive measure, it can take up to three months for this gentle natural substance to work its way into the system fully and start to produce results. For those of us who have been weakened by long-term or chronic sickness, it can take longer. Taking a higher dosage than normal can help to speed up the effects of the therapy, but otherwise persistence is the keyword. Within the first two months you should begin to notice some improvements, no matter how small, and these are a sign that eventually royal jelly will bring you greater benefits.

One other thing should be noted, and this is that during the first few days of your treatment you may actually feel worse. Royal jelly acts as a cleanser, helping the body to eliminate all wastes and toxins produced by the illness. As these toxins are cleared through the system and removed once and for all, your symptoms may get briefly worse. However, this only takes a few days at most, and then your body is free of all the poisonous by-products of the illness. This leaves you much more capable of being healed, so the brief period of worsening is not really a drawback.

Royal jelly is a simple, safe and effective treatment which is fully compatible with all other therapies. It is widely available through health food shops and chemists, but be careful which brand you buy. They are not all equally effective. When I am asked to recommend the best I always suggest Regina Royal Jelly Ltd. The royal jelly in their products is pure, fresh and unprocessed. It comes only from beehives situated in remote regions of China where the air is pure and the crops are free of poisonous insecticides and fertilizers. If you have any difficulty in buying Regina products in your area, you can write to the manufacturers to find out the address of your local stockist or importer. Alternatively, you can order a supply of royal jelly directly from the company. The address of Regina Royal Jelly Ltd can be found in the resource section at the end of this book.

At the time of writing Regina are carrying out medical trials of their royal jelly products against M.E. So far all of the trial participants have noted benefits of one sort or another and there is generally a feeling of great optimism that by the end of the trial some great improvements will have occurred. The trial participants are all impressed with their own responses to the royal jelly treatment. This, plus my own experience with royal jelly, leads me to recommend it unreservedly to all sufferers from M.E. If you would like to try royal jelly, drop a line to the company to find out the results of the trial. They will be able to send you more information about royal jelly and to suggest which of their products would be most suitable for use in your particular case. When the trial has ended, they will also be able to tell you what is the most effective dosage, and so forth.

Tissue salts

Tissue salts, or biochemic remedies as they are more formally known, were developed by Dr Wilhelm Schuessler in the last century. The remedies are each composed of a natural mineral which is necessary for proper functioning of cells in the human body.

The theory that deficiencies of minerals in the cells could cause an overall disturbance of health became the life's work of Dr Schuessler. His research led to the discovery of five principles:

1. Disease does not occur if cell activity is normal.
2. Cell activity is normal as long as all necessary nutrients are available.
3. The human body requires minerals as cell nutrients.
4. Mineral deficiencies will prevent the cell from functioning normally.
5. Individual cells, and therefore the whole metabolism, can be revitalized by correcting mineral deficiencies.

The doctor isolated twelve minerals which are necessary for health, and used the homoeopathic principle of trituration to form tablets which included a tiny dose of each mineral. All of the twelve tissue salts are completely safe and can be taken alone or in combination with other salts or therapies without any fear of side-effects.

In this therapy it is the predominant symptoms which point to the salt or salts necessary. For M.E. sufferers, for example, tissue salt number 6 (Kali Phos) is indicated in cases of nervous tension, depression and general debility; whereas muscular weakness would suggest the use of tissue salt number 1 (Calc Fluor). In addition to these two remedies, tissue salt number 4 (Ferr Phos) relieves muscular pain, and number 10 (Nat Phos) can help in thrush and *Candida* infections. The other salts may be suitable for individuals, but the four mentioned are reliable aids for the majority of M.E. sufferers.

The benefit of this therapy is its simplicity and availability. The tablets can be bought in almost all health shops and in an increasing number of chemists. The tablets are easy and pleasant to take, but you should follow the instructions carefully.

The drawback of this therapy is that lengthy treatment may be necessary before improvements are noticed, especially if your condition is chronic or you have been ill for years. Of course, a speedy reaction to the treatment is possible, but for most people I think it is best to consider this as another background therapy.

Continued treatment often brings relief in the long term, but in the meantime it is best to explore other therapies as well for more immediate benefits.

Vitamins and diet supplements

Several newspapers have reported stories of M.E. sufferers recovering by taking large doses of one vitamin or another. Those who experience dramatic recoveries with this therapy seem to be a very small minority, but it does have a helpful effect on most sufferers.

Unless we have a perfectly balanced diet every day, from time to time we all suffer from shortages of vitamins. There is no doubt that this is harmful if it continues over a long period of time. For M.E. patients this is one more thing that can provoke illness, even in the short term. Vitamins are essential for the proper functioning of all bodily systems. Without them, even for a short period, the body is weakened considerably and can no longer defend itself properly against any illness. Making sure that your intake of food includes sufficient vitamins is a simple way to ensure that your body has everything it needs to function efficiently.

If your diet includes plenty of fresh foods (fruit, vegetables, meat, fish, etc.) which have not been processed or overcooked, then in all probability you are getting an adequate supply of vitamins. As an insurance it is a good idea to take a daily multi-vitamin capsule. These can be bought from any health food shop or chemist.

Some people, myself included, have found it helpful to take a greater than normal amount of certain vitamins – particularly vitamin C and the B group, especially B_6. It is possible that M.E. somehow increases your need of these vitamins, and it is quite safe to take them regularly. A good way to boost your vitamin B intake is to take a daily supplement of brewers yeast, but take care. If you suffer from thrush or other *Candida* problems this may cause difficulties, and in this case you should try a yeast-free supplement instead.

Recent research in Canadian hospitals indicates that the vast majority of all illnesses can be helped by increasing the patient's intake of vitamin C. The researchers gave every patient in a certain hospital high daily doses of this vitamin, and monitored their progress, compared with patients in another hospital who received no additional vitamins. The results were quite amazing. Relief from all sorts of problems was recorded, and recovery times were cut dramatically. This confirms the growing amount of evidence that high doses of vitamins can have an extraordinary effect on the body. In past experiments, even cancer patients and people suffering from other incurable diseases have responded incredibly well to this therapy. This suggests that anyone who is experiencing illness would do well to keep a close eye on their vitamin intake. However, extremely high doses of vitamins should only be experimented with under the supervision of a qualified physician.

Minerals, too, are necessary for a healthy body, but in much smaller amounts than vitamins. Certain minerals can be lacking from your diet for any number of reasons, including your geographical location. Making sure that your diet is supplemented with minerals, or trace elements as they are called, is a sensible preventive measure. Multi-mineral tablets are freely available, and can often be bought combined with multi-vitamins. This simplifies the whole therapy into a one-tablet-a-day regime.

There is a growing awareness that minerals can have a dramatic effect on health. Two minerals in particular have been mentioned in connection with M.E. Germanium and selenium are currently being researched quite extensively because there is reason to believe that they strengthen the body's immune system, helping it to heal itself of disease. Trials have been carried out using these substances, and although the results are not always conclusive, they do suggest that in some cases a daily dose of one of these minerals can promote a speedy recovery. As long as you follow the dosage instructions carefully, these diet supplements should be perfectly safe, so it may be worthwhile for you to try them. However, these immune-supportive substances are a relatively new approach to treatment and as yet we do not know exactly how or why they work. If you think that an immune-supportive supplement is a good idea, I would suggest that you try royal jelly first. As I have already noted, royal jelly supports the immune system in many ways, and it has been thoroughly researched. We know that it is perfectly safe, and as well as strengthening the immune system it provides essential vitamins and minerals in an easily absorbable form. Royal jelly is the finest and best established immune-supportive supplement currently available.

A number of other diet supplements have been tried by M.E. patients. In some cases they report substantial improvements, while in others there is no improvement at all. As the response to these supplements is so varied, I cannot really recommend them fully. However, they seem to suit some people admirably, so it may be a good idea to give them a short trial. If you have tried any of these supplements before for other ailments and found them successful, that is a good indication that they will probably help you to some extent in combating M.E.

The first of these possible therapies is Evening Primrose Oil. It is often sold as a remedy for pre-menstrual tension, but do not let that put you off. It seems to be beneficial in a number of ways, including having a strengthening and balancing effect on the nervous system, so this remedy may be helpful against the nervous disorders associated with M.E. Most people who have tried it continue to take it regularly, which is some indication that it is doing them good, but often they cannot put their finger on any specific improvement.

Ginseng is one of the more popular diet supplements. I have heard it praised quite highly, but again the people who like it find it difficult to express exactly what is improved by it. As it is generally known for its tonic properties, it is reasonable to assume that it will harmonize the body, allowing it to heal itself more effectively. I would imagine that it also boosts your energy reserves, and so may be an antidote to the weakness and tiredness which affects so many sufferers.

Garlic, both fresh and encapsulated, is another remedy which has achieved a degree of popularity. It is usually prescribed for problems of the heart, lungs or digestive system, so quite how it affects M.E. is a mystery. Again, the improvements it brings tend to be minor, but some sufferers, particularly those with predominantly muscular symptoms, find it beneficial as a regular supplement. They recommend that it should be taken in high doses, so it might be just as well to protect your social life by taking the deodorized capsules rather than the fresh plant.

Shark Liver Oil is a relatively new product to come on to

the market. As yet its properties are not fully understood, but there are claims that is a powerful immune-supportive agent. It has been used in trials against certain types of cancer with some impressive results, but this research is definitely in its infancy. It will be many years before it is fully documented. M.E. patients who have tried this supplement are quite complimentary about it, reporting a general all-over lightening of symptoms. The degree of relief varies significantly from person to person.

All of the diet supplements mentioned here are safe to use as a regular daily therapy. It is worth experimenting further in this field, to try to discover a supplement that really gives you a boost, but do not be disappointed if you have only minor successes. In most cases, diet supplements should be thought of as a background therapy.

Yoga

Yoga can best be defined as the science of maintaining a healthy mind in a healthy body, and it has always been known as a preventive therapy. Increasingly, it is also being used in a remedial way to produce cures or alleviation of disease. Research in India and elsewhere has identified specific areas in which yoga practice, particularly hatha yoga, can reliably produce alleviation of illness. In many cases it leads to permanent cures. Some of these areas are very relevant to M.E. sufferers – constipation, migraine, neck and back pain, nervous debilitation and depression.

Yoga is basically a philosophy, a way of thinking and a way of life. It embraces every aspect of existence, spiritual, emotional, mental and physical. It is a system of conscious evolution or self-improvement which has been cherished and embellished over the 6000 years of its documented existence. The main reasons why people take up yoga are to reduce nervous tension, to slim or to become more agile physically and mentally. However, a study of yoga leads naturally to meditation, modifications of thought and behaviour and a new realization of the purposes and processes of life. This holistic approach leads to better health and the eradication of physical and mental dis-ease.

The belief underlying yoga is that most ailment͜
by wrong posture, wrong diet and wrong mental attitu͜
imbalances are under the control of the student, o͜
exclusively and only they can correct them. Therefor͜
to the student to improve their own lot by regular and ͜ ͜per
practice of yoga techniques. The therapist, or teacher, is not
in any way responsible for the student's success or failure. They
are only there to help the student learn the techniques correctly,
and to suggest which of the techniques might be most suitable
in any given situation. Responsibility for the success of the
therapy lies entirely with the student.

A typical hatha yoga class consists of exercises performed
standing, kneeling, sitting, lying on the back, lying on the front
and inverted. The exercises are performed slowly and gently,
and should never cause any undue effort or strain. The aim
of the exercises is to strengthen and improve the flow of subtle
energies by flexing the whole body and by holding certain
postures. Any strain or effort is counter-productive as it can
weaken or block the energy flows rather than strengthening
them. Along with the exercises the class will probably include
a number of relaxation intervals, in which the students are taught
to relax completely, or perhaps an introduction to meditation.

After a properly conducted yoga session you should feel
relaxed and at peace, both mentally and physically, with no
subsequent pains from over-exertion, nor should you have any
feeling of having performed well or badly compared with the
other students. Yoga is totally uncompetitive. You go as far with
each exercise as you comfortably can, and no further. As you
master each posture and become able to perform it easily, the
teacher will introduce you to a new exercise or a new variation
on the one you are doing, so that you are constantly putting
the best effort you can muster into a series of increasingly taxing
postures.

For M.E. sufferers, yoga is partially exempt from the general
rule of avoiding physical exercise. Under the guidance of an
experienced teacher, yoga is probably safe for even a complete
beginner who suffers from this disease. Experienced students
with M.E. can continue their practices, but should be prepared
to drop back to simple exercises or to give up altogether during
bouts of illness. As always, remain highly aware of your own

state of health, and discontinue any exercises which affect you adversely.

One of the breath control, or *pranayama*, exercises of yoga is excellent for all ill people, regardless of the nature of their ailment. It aids breathing, circulation and digestion, and prevents constipation. It produces deep relaxation and mental clarity, removing all fatigue and tension. It is also perfectly safe for daily, or more frequent use.

Sit or lie in a comfortable position, making sure that your chest and stomach can move freely. Keeping your mouth closed, breathe in through your nostrils. Breathe in until your lungs are comfortably full of air and your stomach is pushed out. Then breathe out, pulling your stomach in until your chest deflates. Repeat this a few times to get the feel of it. Remember to breathe slowly and evenly, keeping your mouth closed.

Once you have got the feel of this deep breathing, start to count mentally while you breathe. Count slowly to 4 while you breathe in. Then hold your breath for the same count, by holding the muscles of your chest and stomach quite still. Then breathe out to a count of 6, and again hold the muscles of your chest and stomach still for a count of 4. Then repeat the whole exercise again, starting with the in breath. Continue for as long as you like, but always try to keep it going for at least several minutes. Remember to breathe evenly and slowly, and never hold your breath by closing the throat; keeping the muscles of the chest and stomach still will prevent any air entering or leaving your lungs in a much more harmonious fashion.

This regular, rhythmic breathing is an excellent therapy. As you become more experienced with it and do not have to concentrate so hard on the counting, you will be able to feel the relaxation it produces. Five minutes of controlled breathing leaves you refreshed and reinvigorated. When the rhythm of it has become easy to follow, you will find that you can do it at any time and in any situation, and it will always release a new flow of energy into your mind and body.

5

M.A. BEATS M.E.:
the importance of
mental attitude

The workings of the human mind are subtle and little known. We can only guess at the connections between mind and body, and at how these two aspects of self influence each other. The more we learn, the more it seems that mind and body are not two separate things. They form an indivisible whole, like the two sides of a coin. For as long as life lasts mind and body are part of each other, acting and reacting as a single unit.

Accepting this truth about our basic nature means that we have to reconsider our attitudes towards health and illness. Neither of these states can be considered purely physical any longer. We have to realize that physical disease is always accompanied by, and is sometimes caused by, mental dis-ease. Therefore any attempt to cure disease of the body must include curing dis-ease of the mind as well.

Your own mind can be your strongest ally or your greatest enemy in the quest for well-being. If your thought patterns are of health, strength and optimism, your body will be influenced to respond with increased vitality, healing itself rapidly and well. If your thought patterns are despairing, fearful and pessimistic, every healing mechanism in your body will be sabotaged and true health can never be achieved. Learning to harness the power of your own mind and to direct it into positive channels of health and growth is the quickest, safest method of preventing or curing any ailment.

The importance of mental attitude cannot be overstressed. Thinking the right things in the right way is the key to success in any situation. When the situation is illness and your own body is the monitor showing your success or lack of it in no uncertain terms, thinking correctly becomes a necessity rather than an optional extra. Too many people elect to remain unaware of their mental potential, accepting their mental habits and processes as an unchangeable facet of their being, completely beyond control. But in just the same way that your body is always changing, functioning well or badly according to what you put into it, your mind is constantly changing too, adjusting its functions according to the diet of thoughts, ideas and expectations you feed it. Just as an adequate supply of good food will build an efficient and healthy body, an adequate supply of good thoughts will build an efficient and healthy mind. The healthy mind, one free of dis-ease, is a powerful influence to help you overcome bodily disease. The diet of thoughts your mind needs to perform this healing is generally known as positive thinking.

Positive thinking releases a flow of energy into your mind and body. You feel stronger, healthier, more relaxed and more optimistic. If you persist in training your mind to follow positive thought patterns, the cumulative effect is enormous. You can literally feel yourself rising above the pain and weakness of disease. It is like rising up through the rain and clouds into a realm of pure air and sunshine.

Training yourself to think positively is fairly simple but it does require persistence. Every time you feel yourself slipping into a negative attitude you have to make the effort to correct your thoughts, always concentrating on the positive, pleasant alternative. Instead of giving in to fears about your illness, you constantly consciously reinforce your hope: that you are getting better. Instead of feeling miserable because you cannot do the things you want to, concentrate on all of the things that you can do and allow yourself to feel pleasure at each small achievement. If you always make yourself look for the bright side of things you will soon find that no matter how depressing the situation, if you look at it in the right way you can get something positive from it to keep your thoughts on the right track.

There are a few basic rules of positive thinking that you have to abide by if you want your mind to help you. The first is that it is useless to phrase a positive thought in a negative way. For instance, thinking 'I am not ill' will have very little effect at all because it is stressing a negative, 'I am *not* ill.' The same idea expressed positively would probably come out as, 'I am well' or 'I am getting better.' Both of these will have a good effect because they are simple, direct, positive suggestions that your mind can take up and work on.

Another rule, and a very important one, is to let your imagination in on the act. When you tell yourself, 'I am getting better', reinforce this by imagining how great life will be when you are healthy. Imagine yourself strong and alert, free of all symptoms, able to live a happy, healthy, normal life. It does not matter whether you imagine this in pictures or words or feelings or a combination of all of them, as long as you add all the details that are particularly relevant to you. If the thing you miss most is playing squash or golf, you should imagine yourself on the court or fairway having a wonderful time. Whatever you most want to be able to do again should be the central focus of your imaginings, but do not forget the important little things as well – taking a stroll with someone special, visiting friends in the evening or having your family over to dinner. All of these things can be strong sources of positive thought.

The third and final basic rule is to let your emotions run riot. When you have imagined yourself healthy and able, think for a moment about how you are going to feel when you achieve it. Will you feel happy, triumphant, ecstatic, fulfilled? Let your emotions colour in the picture you have imagined, then watch it come to life. Your emotions are the power-house of your mind. Positive thinking provides images of the reality that you are bringing into being, but it is positive feeling which fuels the process of change, moving you towards whatever you have imagined.

On a daily basis you should practise two types of positive thinking. The first type, which I have described above, is very quick and pleasurable to do. Take a few minutes in the morning and a few at night to imagine and feel yourself healthy. After the first few days, when you have got used to the technique and can really get into the 'feel' of what you are doing, you will probably find that just the act of imagining health makes you feel better. Of course, the effects will build up day by day, becoming stronger and more real for as long as you keep thinking positively.

The second type requires more effort and does not produce such noticeable results, but it is effective in the long run and is a necessary support for the first type. It simply consists of being aware of your own thoughts. During bouts of illness it is very easy to slip into bad thought patterns. Simple things like washing-up, making the beds or going shopping can become impossible, and it is natural to regret the fact that you cannot do any of these things.

If you listen carefully to your thoughts at this point, you will probably hear yourself saying something like, 'Oh, I wish I could do that', or, 'I just can't do it. I feel too ill.' As I have said, these regretful thoughts are natural in that situation, but they are also very harmful. By repeating these sort of thoughts you are reinforcing the ideas of 'I can't' and 'I am too ill.' When you find yourself in the middle of thoughts like these you must stop them immediately and replace them firmly with a more positive command, such as, 'I will be able to do that soon' or 'I am getting stronger every day.' After a while, your unconscious mind will get the message that negative thoughts and negative phrases are unwelcome and it will start to present ideas in more positive forms.

When this happens you know that your new, more positive phrasing of ideas has sunk down into the lowest levels of your mind. It is when your unconscious starts habitually thinking in positive ways that you get the most striking results. The two types of positive thinking described here work together to ensure that your unconscious rapidly accepts new thought patterns that will work to your benefit.

There is one other technique of positive thinking that is very simple and effective: the affirmation. Detailed books have been written about this single technique, but in essence it boils down to this – pick a positive, simple slogan for yourself and repeat it as often as possible. I am sure that everyone must have heard of the famous slogan, 'Every day in every way I am getting better and better.' This is a brilliant example of affirmation. It is a short, uncomplicated positive thought expressed in simple terms. Incidentally, it makes a fine affirmation for M.E. patients, but you may prefer to create one tailored to your own specific needs. Ideally an affirmation should express the essence of everything you want your mind to help you achieve. Then regular repetition pushes the idea firmly into your mind at a level where it will influence you deeply. It is usually best to let your emotions help with the affirmation by 'feeling' the meaning of the phrase once a day. Then repeat it to yourself, physically or mentally, every time you find yourself sliding backwards into doubt or negativity.

Some people think that the simple addition to your affirmation routine described below vastly improves results. As I have never tried it, I cannot really comment one way or another except to say that it is based on very sound principles, so it may well be worth your while to try it if you get on well with the standard affirmation technique. There is no generally accepted name for this technique, but I have always known it as the affirmation spot.

The affirmation spot is very simple to make and use. Get yourself a small piece of paper or card, and on one side colour in a circle of about a ¼-inch diameter. Use a nice bright colour for the spot – red is ideal. When you have finished, select a time and place which you know will be peaceful, so that you will be uninterrupted for five minutes while you 'charge' the spot.

Charging the spot is simplicity itself. Just look at it while you think of your affirmation. Say it to yourself mentally and physically, repeating it over and over again. Let your emotions feel the meaning of your slogan. Imagine how life will be when your affirmation has become reality. Try to make it an intensely positive experience. When you have finished, all that remains to be done is to put your affirmation spot in a place where you will see it fairly frequently. By the kettle or sink would perhaps be a good place for you, or over a mirror or on a coffee table. If you are at work, place the spot on a door or inside a drawer – anywhere where you will see it at least three or four times a day will be fine.

The principle of this technique is that when charging the spot you are concentrating on the simple image of the coloured circle, driving this image deep into your mind. Along with the image go all of the thoughts and feeling conjured up by the affirmation. Afterwards, every time you see the spot you are reminded of the intense positive thought you charged the spot with. This keeps your conscious mind working along the positive track expressed in the affirmation. More importantly, it continually prompts your unconscious, acting as a command to speed and strengthen the healing process. Recharging your spot once a week or so will maintain a high level of effectiveness.

Apart from the direct benefits to health of positive thinking, there are other desirable side-effects. The most important of these is a renewal of your self-respect. Long-term illness can make you feel like a waste of space, a millstone around your family's necks. Thinking positively helps you adjust to the fact that you are to some extent reliant on others. Adjusting to this fact well takes a lot of pressure off you and the people who care for you, and allows everyone to be more optimistic.

Having the support of your family and friends is a very necessary thing. When you are in a bout of illness, they may be your only link with the world outside your illness. Even when you are convalescent and able to get out and about on your own, the people around you are a valuable source of news, gossip and entertainment which keeps you in touch with normality. They are a breath of fresh air in a world which may have shrunk to the size of your own house or room.

Spare a thought occasionally for your carers, because they are doing an extremely difficult job. They have watched you change from a normal human being into a withdrawn, unresponsive, dependent patient. Watching someone you care for going through a disease like M.E. is a frightening experience. You instinctively want to protect your loved one, but there is absolutely nothing you can do to ease their pain. Very often the carers are as frustrated by the illness as the patient is.

Over a period of time this frustration can wear down the carers' understanding to the point where they seem to become unsympathetic. The constant pressure of not knowing what to do or how to help becomes unbearable, and they would rather not be around the illness, and therefore the patient, any more. Turning away from the reality of the situation like this does relieve the pressure of helplessness, but it puts even greater pressure on the relationship between you if the carers have retreated emotionally.

It is your job as the patient to help your carers whenever and however possible. Obviously, when you are very ill there is little you can do to make their job easier. In convalescence, however, you must make every effort to support the people who are supporting you. The most vital thing is to communicate with them. You may feel that you have little or nothing of interest to say, but say it anyway. Talking, even if it is only about the weather, reassures your carers that you are back in the land of the living. Tell them how your day has been, concentrating on all of the little achievements. Talk with them about the news, or a book you are reading, or their interests or hobbies. Always make the effort to chat. It is the most basic form of human communication and it is immensely comforting to all concerned.

Another way in which you can help your carers is to accept their support gracefully. It is very easy to get into the habit of feeling guilty about the demands and pressures you are putting on the people around you. This guilt stems from a feeling of inadequacy – you cannot do for yourself the things which you think you should be doing. Feeling this way can lead to your rejecting the help that people offer, or even to rejecting the people themselves. This creates a very bad atmosphere. For everyone's sake you must learn to overcome this guilt and treat your carers with the respect and courtesy that they deserve.

If people offer to help you with things that you cannot do for yourself, accept the help gracefully and always express your thanks to them. If you find yourself getting caught up in feelings of guilt about accepting aid, tell yourself firmly that you need help at the moment but you will soon be well enough to take care of yourself. This is not only good positive thinking, it is good practical thinking too. You get the help you need, which makes you feel better, and your carers are able to express their concern by helping you, which makes them feel better. Remember that your carers are as frustrated by your illness as you are, and helping you is the only way in which they can feel as if they are doing something constructive to ease your situation.

Apart from the support offered by friends and relatives, some people find that sufferers' groups can be very helpful. As the name implies, these are local groups of sufferers who get together once in a while to compare notes and talk about anything relevant to M.E. Meeting other sufferers is usually a very good thing. You no longer feel so dreadfully alone in your fight against the illness, and there is a sense of camaraderie amongst sufferers which can be the basis of some very good friendships.

Unfortunately, there can also be a negative element about these groups which is harmful. Some groups seem to consist of sufferers who focus exclusively on the pains and problems of the illness, which can be immensely depressing. Most groups, though, approach the subject with a sense of humour, helping the sufferers to laugh at themselves and find the bright side of difficult situations. These groups are also an excellent way of keeping in touch with any new developments in research or treatment, as well as providing a good source of tried and true tips on how to cope with the various aspects of the illness.

This exchange of information is the most important thing that goes on in sufferers' groups. Other sufferers can always suggest therapies and techniques which you may find helpful, or tell you of energy-saving ways to go about necessary tasks. This makes you feel as though you have some ammunition with which to fight the disease, and that helps to keep you optimistic. Another benefit is that you always find people who have individual symptoms much more severely than you do, and this helps you to keep things in perspective and on a positive track.

Often the most valuable advice a newcomer receives from longer-term sufferers is this: learn your own limitations. This is the most basic rule of living with M.E., and you ignore it at your peril. You must try to develop an attitude of constant awareness of your energy levels, and as soon as they start to drop to a degree where your symptoms could get worse, you must rest immediately. This regime of limitation can get incredibly frustrating, but if you do not enforce it, then the virus will, by making you ill every time you deplete your energy reserves.

Living within the limits of your resources demands that you adopt an attitude that borders on selfishness. If you are out shopping, or in the middle of cooking dinner or entertaining friends when you feel your energy drop, you have to stop immediately and have a rest. Many sufferers intensely dislike being self-centred in this way. They consider that they are already causing enough problems for their friends and families without stopping dead in the middle of an outing or chore. However, it is necessary that you do this when the need arises, so you must make up your mind to accept it as a temporary fact of life.

It helps if you stop thinking of this behaviour as self-centred, and start thinking of it in terms of 'centred-with-self'. This might seem like word play and of little practical value, but in fact it does help. By using the term 'centred-with-self', you are removing all of the selfish, 'me first' connotations that we associate with the term 'self-centred'. 'Centred-with-self' is simply an acknowledgement that for a while you must put your own needs first. Putting your own needs first will, of course, work to everyone's benefit in the long run. By protecting yourself in the present you are preventing relapses and future complications that could keep you ill and disabled for months.

Whilst it is very important to live sensibly and stay well within the bounds of your strength, it is also necessary that you do whatever you can. You may often find yourself in a situation where you are feeling up to doing something, but know that you will not have the stamina to finish the job. You might find yourself thinking, 'If I can't finish it, then it's not worth starting.' This is an understandable attitude but a bad one. Always do the maximum that you safely can. If that means starting a job one day and finishing it the next, or the day after, that is fine. Making yourself do little bits and pieces has several good effects. The first is that the physical exercise, as long as it is not too strenuous, will act as a tonic, helping your body to function efficiently. The second and most important effect is that the exercise will tone up your mind and give you a little glow of satisfaction at having achieved something. This helps you to stay positive and to maintain a healthy self-respect.

Every little thing that you can do should act as a trigger for you to indulge in a little self-satisfaction. Think of all the little things as stepping-stones back to health, each one bringing you a little closer to the day when you will be fully active. Use these little achievements to reinforce your positive thinking, keeping your thoughts firmly centred on health rather than illness.

Remember also to keep things in perspective. If you have been so ill that making a cup of tea seemed like a lifetime's work, then this has ceased to be a trivial thing. The first time you make a cup of tea without really thinking about it is a massive achievement, comparable to running a marathon or passing your driving test. Congratulate yourself on this big step forward, allow yourself to feel pleased and satisfied, and celebrate by getting out the sticky buns to go with this momentous cuppa.

When you have only enough energy to do one thing per day, what should it be? The washing-up? Spending time with your family? Taking a short walk? If you can decide what to do then you have decided what your priority is and you should stick to it. Many of the things that we wish we could do in the course of a day are really very unimportant, so it is wise to decide what deserves your best efforts. Getting your priorities in order is a good way to ensure that you do not waste the little energy you have on meaningless pursuits. Look ahead to identify each day's major items, and plan your activities so that you are rested and refreshed when something important is coming up. This will make you feel that you are coping with life more successfully, and that you are responding well to those things that most require your time and energy.

All of the things I have talked about in this chapter are to do with attitude. Developing the right attitude to your illness will reduce your suffering, make life easier for you and your carers and result in a quicker recovery. The wrong attitude will have exactly the reverse effect, and can undo much of the good done by any therapies you may try. Your thoughts are very powerful things within the confines of your body. Make sure that this power is working with you, not against you.

6

FOR THE CARERS

As I have already pointed out, watching a close friend or loved one going through a disease like M.E. is a trying experience. In the early stages, both patient and carer are frightened and worried about the cause of this ailment. Just as the patient unconsciously fears a fatal or degenerative disease, so do you, the carer. In this sense an accurate and speedy diagnosis is just as important for you as it is for the sufferer. During the later stages of the illness, the pressures on the patient tend to remain fairly constant, whereas the carer's pressures change and grow.

If you live with a sufferer, in the first few weeks and months of the illness the greatest pressures on you are going to be the practical ones – shouldering the burden of shopping, housework, cleaning, cooking and all of the other activities that used to be performed jointly or by the sufferer alone. At first this extra work-load is not too much of a problem. In a way, doing all of these extra tasks expresses your desire to help your disabled mate, spouse, parent or offspring. In time, however, the burden can become very heavy indeed. You may be working to support the family, taking care of children and maintaining a home, and far from offering any support or assistance, the sufferer is just another responsibility, another demand upon your resources. Over a period of months, or even years if the illness is severe, you can find your sympathy and supportiveness ebbing away completely.

This practical burden is complicated by the emotional burden of the illness. When the sufferer is too ill to understand you or respond to you in any way, you will feel totally cut off from them and totally unappreciated. When the sufferer is experiencing mood swings or depressions, you will feel unsure how to handle this new and strange personality. When the sufferer is in pain, confused and frustrated by their own weakness, you will bear the brunt of their anger, guilt and inadequacy. And overriding all this is the constant helplessness of not being able to make things better. In this situation it would not be at all surprising if you started to feel that you needed to get away from the illness, and away from the person who is putting such demands upon you. But getting away can make you feel guilty of desertion.

Many marriages in which one partner is a sufferer have almost come to grief over this thorny problem. Maintaining high levels of care and sympathy for the helpless patient who was once your spouse is nearly impossible, without certain adjustments. The major adjustment the carer must make is exactly the same as the one that must be made by the sufferer: learning to live with M.E.

Just as the sufferer must make adjustments to their physical lifestyle, so must the carer: you must allow more time for those extra chores, plan your time and energy wisely and decide what are priorities and what can wait. Just as the sufferer must make adjustments to their mental attitudes and processes, so must the carer: you must learn to think positively, maintain a degree of optimism and keep things in perspective. Just as the sufferer must make adjustments to their emotional responses, so must the carer: you must learn to release negative feelings, focus on the good feelings accompanying every small achievement and consciously reinforce the image of a normal, happy, healthy lifestyle.

This whole book is about helping sufferers to find the breathing spaces which help them to get away from the illness in order to refresh their minds and bodies. You, as the carer, must also allow yourself the time to get away from the illness. Regularly pursuing your favourite sport or hobby is an excellent way to forget the illness for a while. Never feel guilty about going out and having fun when your sufferer is ill at home. Making sure that you do forget all about the illness whenever you need to is good for everyone concerned. You will return to the sufferer refreshed in mind and body, more willing and able to care for them in a spirit of sympathy. Equally, the sufferer will feel less guilty about being a burden on you. Tying yourself completely to the sufferer for twenty-four hours a day is the fastest way to wear yourself down utterly, destroying the strength and resilience that both of you need badly. Consciously plan ahead to set aside fun times for yourself, to get away from all the limitations of M.E.

Any of the therapies mentioned in this book will be excellent for you to use as a preventive measure, safeguarding your own well-being. Also, learning about and practising the therapies can become a fun time for both of you to participate in. This shared activity will be beneficial to the health of both of you, and will also help to maintain the bonds of togetherness and shared experience which help to keep all relationships growing. Going to see a healer together, or taking your royal jelly capsules every morning, or learning to meditate or experimenting with aromatherapy – all these enhance the bond between you and help to keep your relationship stable in spite of the illness.

These shared activities can be a lifeline for the sufferer. After being isolated for weeks by a thick fog of pain and confusion, hating themself for being so feeble, having someone there who understands the limitations and can take them out of themself for a while is wonderful. Once, when I was just coming out of a particularly bad bout of illness, a friend arrived one morning to take me on a so-called mystery tour. In fact, there was not much mystery about it because she took me to some local woodland that I had known for years. She knew, though, that I had also loved it for years and that being there in the fresh air had always been a wonderful therapy for me. We sat and talked in the sunshine for a while, and then she dropped me off at home. I was absolutely exhausted, but it was a good healthy tiredness. I slept well and awoke refreshed. The fact that my friend had involved herself in my therapy, and helped me in a very practical way, was a real tonic. It made me feel as though I had re-established contact with the human race.

Caring for anyone with a long-term or chronic illness is all about keeping up a degree of normality, sharing things in the way you used to. Of course, the things you share will have to change, because of the limitations of the illness, but the act of sharing can and should be maintained. This applies to friends of M.E. sufferers as well as to live-in carers.

If you have a friend who is suffering from this debilitating disease, then you will find your friendship going through a very

tough time. Most friendships are based on the things that people
do together, and there is very little an M.E. patient can do when
ill or convalescing. Many sufferers, particularly those in the
younger age groups, have found that their friends start to
disappear from sight after the first few weeks of illness. This
is unfortunate, but fully understandable. It is during periods
of convalescence and remission when the sufferer is alert enough
to want and need human contact that the lack of friendly visits
and phone calls becomes most noticeable. At this stage it can
be very depressing to feel isolated and out of touch with your
friends.

If you are friendly with a sufferer, please try to make the effort
to stay in touch. A five-minute phone call can make an
extraordinary difference in the sufferer's day. On many occasions
during the course of my illness, I was too well to stay in bed
sleeping, but too ill to do anything interesting or go out. At these
times I would feel bored and listless, trapped inside the walls
of my house. A phone call was then an absolute godsend. The
fact that someone had bothered to pick up the phone to find
out how I was doing and to chat for a few minutes seemed like
a real life-saver, or a sanity-saver at least.

Strangely enough, very often the sufferer does not feel able
to call their friends, no matter how bored or restless they feel.
I can fully sympathize with this. After all, when they call
someone what do they have to say: that they are still feeling
awful and have not been anywhere or seen anyone? It is not
nice to inflict all of this bad news on their friends. They feel
as though they are infecting others with their boredom and
misery. If, on the other hand, others call them, it is much easier
to gloss over their own situation and concentrate on talking about
the callers. Chatting with a healthy friend about their activities
and thoughts can be a real high point in the sufferer's day. It
helps to establish a feeling of normality and contact with the
real world.

Occasional visits are good for the sufferer too, though they
may not be terribly entertaining for the visiting friend. If you
want to visit a suffering friend, your visit will be much
appreciated as long as you do not just turn up out of the blue.
Unless you know quite well how the sufferer is feeling, an
unplanned visit is not always a good idea. If the sufferer is in

a period of illness, they probably need to be left alone. If they are in convalescence, you may turn up when they need to be sleeping or resting. A phone call before you arrive is always a good idea. If you turn up at a bad time it can be awkward for all concerned. If the sufferer is too embarrassed to explain the situation to you and to ask you to leave, it can lead to them over-exerting themself because of your visit. Keeping in touch with the sufferer fairly regularly is the best way to get an idea of the state of their health. You will soon be knowledgeable enough about their pattern of good and bad times to know when a visit would be most welcome.

Finally, the one thing a sufferer needs from the people round about more than anything else is their optimism, their belief that in the not too distant future the sufferer will be back to ruddy health. Because M.E. is a long and severe illness, it is all too easy for the sufferer to lose their sense of direction, their aims and their goals. In effect, they get lost in the illness and can no longer see any possibility of health. Having someone around who believes in their ability to beat the disease is a constant help. It is like a signpost that always points in the right direction, encouraging the sufferer to take the next step, and the next, back to health.

USEFUL ADDRESSES

Myalgic Encephalomyelitis
  Association
PO Box 8
Stanford le Hope
Essex SS17 8EX
(Telephone: 0375 642466)

M.E. Action Campaign
PO Box 1126
London
W3 0RY
(send SAE for information)

Australia

ANZAMES
PO Box 645
Mona Vale
NSW 2103

Canada

Mrs K.M. Smith
PO Box 298
Kleinburg
Ontario
L0J 1CO

Holland

Ms Marion Lescrauwaet
1106 DP Wamelplein 16
Amsterdam

New Zealand

ANZAMES
PO Box 35/429
Browns Bay
Auckland 10

Norway

Ellen Piro
Gullerasveien 14B
0386 Oslo 3

South Africa

Mrs Janine Shavell
66 Third Street
Lower-Houghton
Johannesburg

USA

Chronic Fatigue Syndrome
  Society
PO Box 230108
Portland
Oregon 97223
(Telephone: (503) 684 5261)

Treatment information sources:

Acupuncture
The Council for Acupuncture, Suite 1, 19a Cavendish Square,
  London W1M 9AD.

Aromatherapy
International Federation of Aromatherapists, 46 Dalkeith Road,
  London SE21 8LS.

Autogenic Training
The Positive Health Centre, 101 Harley Street,
  London W1N 1DF.

Bach Flower Therapy
The Edward Bach Centre, Mount Vernon, Sotwell, Wallingford,
  Oxon OX10 0PZ.

Biochemic Tissue Salts
New Era Laboratories Ltd., Marfleet, Hull HU9 5NJ.

Clinical Ecology
The Society for Environmental Therapy, 521 Foxhall Road,
  Ipswich, Suffolk IP3 8LW.

Colonic Irrigation
Colon Hydrotherapy Foundation of Great Britain, 10 Willow
  Walk, Sutton, Surrey.

Healing
Confederation of Healing Organizations, 113 Hampstead Way,
  London NW11 7JN.

Herbal Medicine
National Institute of Medical Herbalists, 41 Hatherley Road,
  Winchester, Hampshire SO22 6RR.

Homoeopathy
British Homoeopathic Association, 27a Devonshire Street, London W1N 1RJ.
Society of Homoeopaths, 2 Artizan Road, Northampton NN1 4HU.

Hypnotherapy
British Hypnotherapy Association, 67 Upper Berkeley Street, London W1.

Kinesiology
The Association of Systematic Kinesiology, 39 Browns Road, Surbiton, Surrey KT5 8ST.

Naturopathy
British Naturopathic and Osteopathic Association, Frazer House, 6 Netherhall Gardens, London NW3 5RR.

Reflexology
British Reflexology Association, Monks Orchard, Whitbourne, Worcester WR6 5RB.

Royal Jelly
Wardglen, Regina House, Elstree Gate, Elstree Way, Borehamwood, Hertfordshire WD6 1JD.

Yoga
British Wheel of Yoga, 80 Leckhampton Road, Cheltenham, Gloucestershire GL53 0BN.

FURTHER READING

Candida Albicans, Leon Chaitow, Thorsons (1985).

The Beat Fatigue Workbook, Leon Chaitow, Thorsons (1988).

Royal Jelly, Irene Stein, Thorsons (1986).

The Miracle Nutrient CoEnzyme Q10, Dr Emile G. Bliznakov and Gerald Hunt, Thorsons (1988).

Germanium: The health and life enhancer, Sandra Goodman Ph.D., Thorsons (1988).

Selenium, Dr Eric Trimmer, Thorsons (1988).

Yoga for All Ages, Cheryl Isaacson, Thorsons (1986).

The Vital Vitamin Fact File, Dr H. Winter Griffith, Thorsons (1988).

Relaxation, Sandra Horn, Thorsons (1986).

Reflexology Today, Doreen Bayly, Thorsons (1982).

Applied Kinesiology, Tom and Carole Valentine, Thorsons (1985).

Autohypnosis, Ronald Shone, Thorsons (1987).

Homoeopathy: Medicine of the new man, George Vithoulkas, Thorsons (1985).

The Dictionary of Modern Herbalism, Simon Mills, Thorsons (1985).

Spiritual Healing: A patient's guide, Eileen Herzberg, Thorsons (1988).

Bach Flower Therapy, Mechthilde Scheffer, Thorsons (1986).

Practical Aromatherapy, Shirley Price, Thorsons (1987).

Acupuncture: A patient's guide, Dr Paul Marcus, Thorsons (1984).

Acupressure Techniques, Dr Julian Kenyon, Thorsons (1987).

INDEX

acupressure, 31, 52-4
acupuncture, 31, 52-4, 77
affirmation, 92-3, 94-6
alcohol, 63
allergies, 38, 63
alternative therapies, 12, 13, 18, 48-90
   and orthodox medicine, 48-9, 50
   philosophy of, 50-1
     see also under individual names
anti-social phases, 47
antibiotics, 10, 11
appetite disorders, 40-1, 63-4
aromatherapy, 56-9, 69, 71, 76, 79
attitude, positive, 91-100, 102
autogenic training, 44, 54-6
autohypnosis, 54, 56, 73-4, 80
aversion, food, 63

Bach, Dr Edward, 59-61
Bach flower remedies, 44, 59-61, 69
balance, lack of, 45-6
baths
   hot, 33, 71-2
   neutral, 72
breathing spaces, 17-19, 102-3

Candida overgrowth, 37-8, 85
   relief of, 62, 84

carer
   breathing spaces for, 102-3
   and emotional burden, 101-2
   and practical pressures, 101
   support for, 96
cause of M.E., 10, 13, 19, 20, 23, 27
'centred-with-self', 98-9
coldness, feelings of, 10, 11, 21, 27, 33
   relief of, 71
colonic irrigation, 61-2
communication
   with carer, 96-7
   with doctor, accurate, 15
compatibility of therapies, 54, 56, 69, 71, 72, 74, 76, 79, 80, 83, 84
comprehension, lack of, 15, 21, 44-5
   improved, 35, 56
confusion, 10, 15, 17, 102
constipation, 39
   relief of, 62, 88
contracting M.E., 20
convalescent periods, 11, 12, 17-18, 21-2, 29, 44, 45, 50
co-ordination, lack of, 45
cravings, 63-4
cycle of illness, 22-3

debilitation, 39
   relief of, 84, 88

depression, 10, 11, 17, 36, 41-3, 102
  relief of, 84, 88
desertion, 102
diagnosis, importance of, 12, 13, 14, 16, 28, 101
diet, 31, 34, 39, 62-5
  supplements, 85-8
digestive disorders, 39
  relief of, 78
doctor
  attitude of, 9, 13, 14, 20
  keeping informed, 15, 48, 69
dreams, 34-5
duration of illness, 20, 21-2

emotional problems, 46-7
  relief of, 58-9, 61
emotions, importance of, 24-5, 93
energy
  flow, 52, 53, 92
  gaining control of own, 55
  and healing, 66-7
  increased, 82
  levels awareness, 22, 23, 30-1
exercise, 30, 31-2, 65-6, 89, 99

fatigue *see* tiredness
feelings, effect of, 23-4
fevers, night, 11, 17, 27, 33-4
  relief of, 58, 71
friends, importance of, 96, 104
frustration, 30, 43, 96, 97, 102

glands, 11, 41
groups, support, 12-13, 14, 97-8
guilt feelings, 97, 102

headaches, 27, 31, 41, 88
healing, 44, 54, 66-8, 79
herbalism, 68-9
holistic approach, 49, 88
homoeopathy, 32, 69-70
hydrotherapy, 36, 70-2, 76, 80
hypnosis, 31, 54, 73-4
hysteria, mass, 19-20

Icelandic disease, 20

imagination, use of, 93
immune depression, 36
  relief of, 87, 88-9
infections, 11, 21, 36-7
isolation, feelings of, 103-4

joint pain, 11, 32

kinesiology, 74-5

lifestyle, limitations on, 22, 23-4, 25
limitations, awareness of, 16-17, 22, 23-4, 98
living with M.E., 16, 29, 30, 35, 42, 45, 56, 98-100, 102

massage, 53, 54, 57, 59, 75-6
M.E. Association, 12-13
M.E. throat, 40
meditation, 74, 76-7, 88, 89
memory loss, 11, 15, 21, 43-4
mineral supplements, 86
mood swings, 21, 46, 102
muscle pain, 11, 21, 31-2
  relief of, 56, 82, 84, 87

nausea, 40
note making, 15, 43

optimism, importance of, 105
orthodox medicine, 48-9, 50
over-exertion, 11, 22, 23, 65-6

pain, 11, 17, 21, 27, 31-2, 102
  -killers, 31, 34
  relief of, 72, 82, 84, 88, 102
pallor, 39-40
pattern of illness, 21-2, 23, 27, 28, 29
photophobia, 41
positive thinking, 25, 91-100, 102
  rules of, 92-3
preventive measures, 50, 51, 88
psychiatric treatment, 9, 14, 20
psychosomatic illness, M.E. as, 9, 10, 20, 27

rash, 10, 11
reflexology, 31, 54, 77-9
relapses, 11, 12, 22, 23, 65-6
relaxation, 22, 31, 32, 54, 55-6, 57, 71, 73-4, 76, 78, 90, 92
    technique, 79-80
relief, temporary, 49, 59
responsibility for self, 55, 78, 89
rest, 22
routine, establishing, 29, 30
Royal Free disease, 19
royal jelly, 44, 80-3, 86-7

Schuessler, Dr Wilhelm, 83-4
Schultz, J.H., 54, 55
self-awareness, importance of, 16, 22, 23-4, 29, 30, 89
self-respect, 18, 96, 99
shared activity, 103
signs of illness, first, 10, 21
sleep disorders, 11, 34-5
    improvement of, 58
strength, increased, 53
stress, 16, 24-5, 37
    relief from, 53, 61, 76
sugar, 37-8, 64
support
    for carers, 96
    of family and friends, 96-7
    groups, 97-8
sweats, 17, 33-4, 35-6, 71
    relief of, 58, 71
swellings, 10, 21, 31
    reduction of, 72
symptoms, 10, 11, 21, 27-47

see also under individual names

talking, importance of, 24, 47, 97
tension relief, 57, 72, 80, 88, 90
test for M.E., 13, 21, 28
thrush, 37-8, 85
    relief of, 84
tiredness, 10, 28-9, 37
    over-tiredness as cause of relapse, 11, 22, 23, 65-6
    relief of, 72, 90
tissue salts, 32, 83-5
treatment, 27-8, 29, 30, 31, 32, 34, 36, 37, 38, 42, 44, 48-90
    choosing, 49-50, 51
    wrong, 9, 11, 14
tremors, 32

urine retention, 40

virus as cause, 13, 19, 20, 27
vision, improved, 53
visits, 104-5
vitality, increased, 53, 58
vitamin supplements, 85-8

weakness, 10, 17, 21, 30-1
    muscle, 11, 30
    relief of, 84
will-power, 29, 30

yoga, 74, 80, 88-90
    breathing technique, 90